# THE
# GOOD
# SKIN
# SOLUTION

Natural Healing for
**Eczema, Psoriasis, Rosacea**
and **Acne**

Shann Nix Jones

**HAY HOUSE**

Carlsbad, California • New York City • London
Sydney • Johannesburg • Vancouver • New Delhi

First published and distributed in the United Kingdom by:
Hay House UK Ltd, Astley House, 33 Notting Hill Gate, London W11 3JQ
Tel: +44 (0)20 3675 2450; Fax: +44 (0)20 3675 2451; www.hayhouse.co.uk

Published and distributed in the United States of America by:
Hay House Inc., PO Box 5100, Carlsbad, CA 92018-5100
Tel: (1) 760 431 7695 or (800) 654 5126; Fax: (1) 760 431 6948 or (800) 650 5115
www.hayhouse.com

Published and distributed in Australia by:
Hay House Australia Ltd, 18/36 Ralph St, Alexandria NSW 2015
Tel: (61) 2 9669 4299; Fax: (61) 2 9669 4144; www.hayhouse.com.au

Published and distributed in the Republic of South Africa by:
Hay House SA (Pty) Ltd, PO Box 990, Witkoppen 2068
info@hayhouse.co.za; www.hayhouse.co.za

Published and distributed in India by:
Hay House Publishers India, Muskaan Complex, Plot No.3, B-2,
Vasant Kunj, New Delhi 110 070
Tel: (91) 11 4176 1620; Fax: (91) 11 4176 1630; www.hayhouse.co.in

Distributed in Canada by:
Raincoast Books, 2440 Viking Way, Richmond, B.C. V6V 1N2
Tel: (1) 604 448 7100; Fax: (1) 604 270 7161; www.raincoast.com

A catalogue record for this book is available from the British Library.

ISBN: 978-1-78180-802-3

Interior illustrations: 100,101, 102 © Helen Elliott

Printed and bound by CPI Group (UK) Ltd, Croydon, CR0 4YY

*I'd like to dedicate this book to our lovely, close-knit community of Chuckling Goat readers and clients, many of whom have generously shared the stories and pictures of their own healing journey with us, enabling us to learn so much.*

*I'm grateful to each and every one of you. Reading your success stories keeps us going on the farm when things get tough. We're moving forward hand in hand, working out this stuff together and learning as we go!*

*Hugs from the barn,*

*Shann*

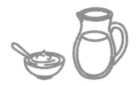

# Contents

## Part III: Understanding Your Skin Disorder

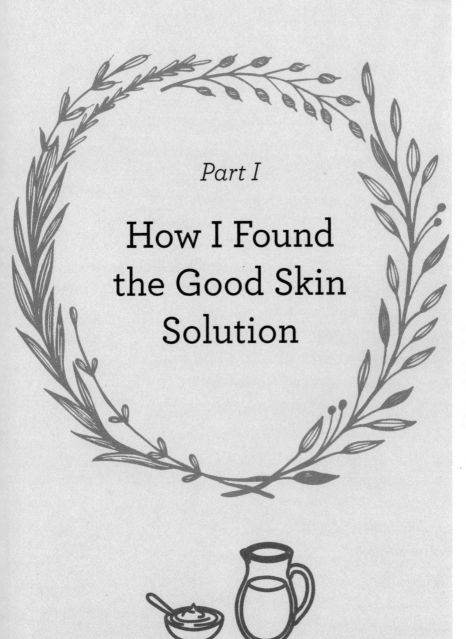

*Part I*

# How I Found the Good Skin Solution

## Chapter 1

# Discoveries

Cameron knocked on the door of the farmhouse at our goat farm in southwest Wales, his other hand clinging tightly to his mum's. When I answered the door, the first thing I noticed was his eyes. Big and dark, they were filled with fierce intelligence.

The next thing I noticed was that he looked absolutely exhausted. Those beautiful eyes were ringed with black, and sunk deep into his skull. I saw, too, that his skin was red and raw-looking, his arms and legs were thin, and his belly was distended. He looked like a little old man. But he was only three years old.

### Cameron's story

Cameron had been suffering from severe eczema since birth. After bathing him, his devoted mum, Michaela, had to lift him out of the bath by his elbows because his entire body was covered with flaming red patches so severe they looked like burns. Neither Cameron nor his mum had slept through an entire night since he'd been born – his itchy, weepy, broken skin kept him in constant torment. And neither of them *ever* had a break.

Michaela had taken her son to every doctor, every hospital, and every consultant she could find, and he'd been prescribed various topical corticosteroids, emollients, antibiotic creams, and ointments... you name it, they had tried it. But nothing had worked.

The last consultant had suggested putting Cameron on immunosuppressants. 'But he's only three. If you suppress his immune system, what will happen next time he catches a virus?' Michaela protested. 'It's a risk,' the consultant admitted. Michaela grabbed Cameron's hand and led him straight out of the consultant's office.

Soon afterwards, desperate for help and advice, Michaela brought Cameron to see us: she'd heard that we'd created some products using the milk from our goats that were proving beneficial for eczema. I invited them in and sat them at our kitchen table, made Michaela a cup of tea and Cameron a cup of goat's milk, and then explained Chuckling Goat's 'Good Skin Solution,' or GSS for short.

**Initially, Michaela was dubious, but with nothing left to lose, she agreed to give the GSS a try. Six months later, Cameron looked like a different boy.**

When I asked Michaela if I could share Cameron's experience in this book, she wrote me the following letter.

## GSS SUCCESS STORY

*Hello, Shann*

*I've bombarded you with photos of Cameron – I just got a bit excited when I looked back and saw how much better he really is! I wanted you to share in this, as without you, who knows where we would be now. Cameron has changed lots. I think he's at the end of his withdrawal from the steroids, and he's so, so active.*

*I mean really, he can at last pedal his toy tractor – it was a big moment for me! He's eating me out of house and home. It's great, except when I run out of ideas for things to cook! He's loving school and thriving there: I can't believe how quickly he's learning things! He's sleeping better at night, too, which is great!*

*I really hope more people will get on the bandwagon for the GSS, and stop using those awful drugs! You've inspired me, and made me see we could get through this: eat well and fight, hope, and just keep going!*

*Thank goodness I wasn't sucked in by the doctors and had the sense to question them. We met you at one of the lowest parts of my life. You really were our saving grace – I will always be so very deeply grateful to you.*

*Love to you all, and the goats.*

**MICHAELA**

(See photographs in the colour section.)

## Looking for answers

So why did Michaela bring Cameron to see me? After all, I'm not a scientist, a doctor, or a faith healer – I'm just a mum and a farmer's wife.

Well, like Michaela, I too had been driven into a corner when doctors were unable to provide answers for medical issues within my family. Determined to save my loved ones, I went in search of my *own* answers – and I was lucky enough to find them.

**Today, I'm in the very fortunate position of being able to share these answers with other people, among them Cameron and his mum. And as a result, in the past few years, *thousands* of people have come to me looking for help with their stubborn eczema, as well as chronic psoriasis, acne, and rosacea.**

You'll read about the experiences of some of these people in the book – I've called them GSS success stories.

But where did these answers come from? Strangely enough, I discovered them in my own farmhouse kitchen.

## From city girl to farmer's wife

Before I moved to Wales from my native United States and married a farmer, I'd enjoyed a long, high-powered career in the media. So when it turned out that in my case, a woman's place really *is* in the kitchen, it came as a huge shock. A controversial one too, I know. But for me personally, it's true.

I've never felt *relegated* to the kitchen; instead, I occupy it as a place of pride. I'm the queen and it's my kingdom – the central hub of the constantly turning wheel of our farm. I experience my position in the farmhouse kitchen as one of power and responsibility.

But, believe me, a Welsh farm was the very *last* place I expected to end up. I was never a domestic person – my mother, who grew up during the feminist revolution, purposefully didn't teach me to cook. She thought that, without those skills, I would be protected from the 'dog work' that women are traditionally expected to do. Freed from that duty by ignorance, she figured, I could go out into the world and have a career instead.

So I did. I spent five years working as a newspaper journalist, 10 years as a San Francisco radio talk show host, and another five years flying all over the world coaching CEOs in the art of communication. My career was my life. Then I went to live in Wales, and fell in love with a Welsh farmer named Rich.

Moving with my two children to live with Rich and his two daughters (and his father, and the boyfriend of one of the older girls), on his beautiful Welsh farm overlooking the sea, was one of the most terrifying steps I've even taken. Suddenly, seven hungry people were staring up at me from the long scrubbed pine table every evening, waiting to be fed. The closest take-out restaurant was a half-hour drive away. So I had to learn to cook – and quickly. And that was only the beginning...

Rich's farm was very nearly self-sustaining – he grew his own hay, raised and butchered his own lambs, made his own beer and cheese. I learned to do these things around the farm as well, along with mucking out stables, helping sheep to give birth, treating sick animals, dealing with death – all the realities of farm life.

It was quite an adventure for a city girl from San Francisco whose biggest previous experience of getting her hands dirty was planting a few begonias in a window box. But to my surprise, when I stepped into the farmhouse kitchen and tied on an apron, I experienced a huge surge of joy and contentment.

## Healing with food

The ancient traditional tasks of bread-making, cooking huge pots of stew, roasting lamb, making cheese, picking berries, and preserving jam filled me with serenity and pleasure. Despite my failures – and believe me, they were many and notable – I loved them all.

Performing the tasks that women have done for thousands of years satisfied something deep inside my DNA. On the day I screwed the top on my first jar of blackberry jam and proudly hand-wrote the label, the ladies in long dresses lining the genetic corridors of my mind all stood and applauded.

The tasks I'd undertaken in my earlier, urban life – whizzing up and down freeways, sitting in plastic cubicles and producing column inches of newspaper copy, or talking into microphones – had never satisfied me in the way this did. This new life on the farm had deep texture, and it filled me up in a totally different way.

Real comfort food, I discovered, was in the *making* of it, not the eating of it. Comfort came from doing. The tasks themselves

– kneading bread, making jam, pressing cheese – made me happy. All of this was a revelation to me.

## Get a goat?!

In 2010, my little boy, Benji, then aged five, began to suffer from severe recurrent bronchial infections. Every time he caught a cold it went straight to his chest, ending in a frightening heavy cough that required antibiotics.

We went to the GP four times in three months, and Benji seemed worse on each occasion. It was clear that his situation was deteriorating, and the antibiotics he'd been prescribed were only making things worse. The condition of Benji's skin appeared to be worsening as well: stubborn patches of eczema had erupted on his hands, inside his elbows, and behind his knees.

I asked Rich what we should do about it. 'Get a goat,' he replied.

Initially, this made no sense to me: how could owning a goat possibly help Benji's bronchial problems? But Rich was aware – from the depths of his own ancient Welsh farming traditions – that goat's milk is good for people with asthma, eczema, and bronchial infections.

By then, I'd been married to Rich long enough to know that he is – annoyingly! – almost always right. We drove straight from the doctor's surgery to see 'a man who had a goat.' There, we paid £50 and brought home the lovely Buddug, a black-and-white Anglo-Nubian goat with long ears and seductive Cleopatra eyes.

I fell in love with Buddug straight away, beginning an enchantment with goats that continues to this day. Buddug was wise, calm, patient – and occasionally entirely mischievous. As I set out to learn how to milk her, she'd look at me sideways and then kick over the milk bucket each time it was nearly full.

I found the goat-milking process hard as hell, and I cried every night during that steep learning curve. But I finally cracked it, and started giving Benji some fresh goat's milk to drink. He loved it. Buddug then began to produce so much milk that very soon, we had a surplus. I felt guilty every time I opened the fridge and saw milk going off, so I learned how to make soap and lotion containing it.

The resulting skincare products were lovely stuff: handmade, all-natural, chemical free, and safe for little ones with sensitive skin. Soon, all the mums on the school run were begging me to make goat's milk skincare for their children. Rich and I bought another goat, and then another, until we owned – and milked – an entire herd.

But we had another issue: making the goat's milk skincare didn't really use up that much milk – I still had loads of it going off in the fridge – so what could we do with the rest?

## We discover kefir

In November 2011, a girlfriend called and excitedly told me to turn on the radio. As I tuned in to the 'Food Show' on BBC Radio 4, I heard Dr. Natasha Campbell-McBride – brilliant creator of the GAPS diet and author of *Gut and Psychology Syndrome: Natural Treatment for Autism, ADD/ADHD, Dyslexia,*

*Dyspraxia, Depression, Schizophrenia* – discussing something called kefir, which she'd recommended to her patients.

She explained that kefir is a powerful probiotic drink made by adding a live culture of yeast and 'good' bacteria to milk and leaving it to ferment for around 24 hours.

Dr. Natasha (as she's known to her grateful patients around the globe) is from Russia, where kefir is drunk every day, so she has long known about its benefits for digestion and gut health. I'd never heard of kefir, and was immediately intrigued. Rich and I contacted Dr. Natasha, and asked for her advice on making kefir properly, in the traditional Russian style, using our goat's milk.

She suggested we use real kefir 'grains' to ferment the milk, rather than powdered kefir 'starter,' which produces a beverage that's far less potent. She also recommended that we keep our kefir unflavored, and avoid adding sugar to it (which compromises the power of the probiotics).

I still remember the amazement I felt after I'd made my first batch of kefir in a kilner jar, and set it to ferment on the windowsill. That was the day I *really* discovered the powerful female tradition of healing with food.

It stunned me to realize that this probiotic medical food could potentially have a profound impact on my family's health. With every choice I made while preparing their meals, I could encourage my family toward wellness, or tilt them toward illness.

Soon, we started making small batches of goat's milk kefir in the little stone outbuilding on our farm. At the time, almost no one in the UK had heard of kefir, and it was a struggle to get people interested in trying it! Our kefir tasted tart, acidic, and fizzy. We left it unflavored, as Dr. Natasha had suggested, so people had to be really convinced of its health benefits before they were willing to buy it.

My son, Benji, was drinking the kefir, and after a while I noticed that it had cleared his asthma, and stopped his cycle of bronchial infections. We put his inhalers away, because he didn't seem to need them anymore.

Terrified but determined, Rich and I both quit our day jobs, and decided to try to make a go of selling our handmade goat's milk products – the drinking kefir and the soaps and lotions – which we had crafted on the farmhouse kitchen table. We packed a few pints of kefir and some of the skincare into the car, drove out to the health food shops in our area, and convinced them to stock our products.

## Starting Chuckling Goat

In the spring of 2011, we launched a small online business; we called it Chuckling Goat, in honor of Buddug, who always seemed to be laughing. Our goat's milk goodies caught on quickly, and by 2012 our business was booming. We bought 20 more goats, and Rich installed a milking machine as a birthday gift to me. I was so excited! No more hauling those heavy stainless-steel milk churns around.

For a while, everything was sunny on our little farm. But then disaster struck...

# How kefir saved my husband's life

In April 2013, my beloved husband, Rich, went into hospital for a major operation, and came out again infected with methicillin-resistant Staphylococcus aureus, or MRSA, an antibiotic-resistant 'superbug.' The 25-cm (10-inch) surgical incision down the midline of his abdomen was contaminated with this flesh-eating horror.

Before long, small red holes appeared down the length of Rich's surgical wound. The district nurse who visited daily began to measure the depths of these holes with a probe, holding them up against a small ruler. Instead of healing, the holes – which looked like angry red mouths – were growing deeper every day.

A doctor was called out to the farmhouse. He peeled back the long bandage on Rich's abdomen and looked at the wound. I watched as the blood drained out of the doctor's face. 'I haven't any experience of something of this magnitude,' he admitted. 'I suggest you contact the surgeon who did the operation.'

I felt stunned. Contact the surgeon? What exactly could he do about a post-operative infection? Operate again? How much could they cut away? How would that possibly help?

Rich had swabbed positive for MRSA, so I guessed the hospital would be reluctant to re-admit him, since they screen for MRSA before admitting patients. Anyhow, Rich had contracted MRSA in the hospital to begin with – and since they didn't have anything to help him, surely he would be better off at home, where at least he wouldn't catch any more cross-infection?

I felt my knees buckle beneath me as I confronted the possibility that, if he couldn't be readmitted to hospital, my husband might actually die on my sofa. Over the next week or so, Rich grew weaker, and kept passing in and out of consciousness. I realized that the day the infection hit his vital organs, our happy ending would be really and truly over.

I gritted my teeth and determined that this was *just not going to happen*; there was no way my husband was going down on my watch. I'd traveled too far, and worked too hard, to find this lovely man when I was 41 years old. This would *not* be the way things ended for us.

## Race against time

Frantically, I began to do research. I uncovered some information suggesting that various combinations of plant-based essential oils might be effective in fighting antibiotic-resistant bacteria. *Essential oils*, I thought, excitedly. *I have loads of those for use in my soaps!*

I hauled out my big stainless-steel saucepan and started experimenting with combinations of essential oils. Eventually, I found a recipe that I thought *might* work to knock back the MRSA levels.

But there was another problem. The surgeon who'd operated on Rich (we *did* contact him in the end, but he too was unable to offer answers) had informed us that MRSA colonizes *all over the body, and not just in the wound itself.*

So, even if I managed to kill off 99 percent of the MRSA cells (all those I could reach, that is), and even if I were to bathe

Rich in pure bleach, there would *still* be a few cells left behind his ears, under his fingernails and so on.

I could *never* kill all the MRSA cells, and those that were left behind would be the strongest, and most resistant, bacteria. Those would survive, re-populate, and just take over again.

How could I fight an enemy that I could never completely eradicate – one that would simply re-grow from any tiny bit I failed to kill? Answer: I couldn't. Result? Loss, failure, death. There was just no winning outcome from that question.

## Asking the right question

And then my Texas-born stubbornness kicked in. It isn't for nothing that I come from a long line of obstinate pioneer women who left their homes behind to launch themselves into the wilderness. I figured that if I didn't like the answer, *I must be asking the wrong question.*

I racked my brain. What *would* be a better question? Not 'How can I fight and kill the MRSA?' Nothing so aggressive would work – and it was that kind of approach that had led to the rise of antibiotic-resistant superbugs in the first place. What about: 'How can the MRSA be *resolved*, and brought into harmony?'

Ah, that was better. With that question, I could begin to see some possible answers. I was looking for resolution, not more death. I needed to create a truce; I needed an ally; I needed a friend on the microbiological level. I had to find something that would help bring the MRSA back under control.

Staphylococcus aureus is a type of bacteria that commonly lives on our skin, and it only becomes a problem when it gets out of balance. So how could I restore that balance?

Well, the one thing I knew restored balance was the kefir we'd been making on the farm. I knew that drinking kefir repopulates the good bacteria living in the gut, and pushes back the pathogens (disease-causing microbes), bringing the system back into balance.

I thought to myself: *What if it works the same way on the skin?* With Rich getting weaker by the day, and without any other options, I figured I had nothing to lose.

First I blended up the special recipe of essential oils I'd come up with after my research. It certainly smelled nice. It couldn't harm Rich, I reasoned, and it just might help him! I put 10 drops of the oil into warm water and bathed Rich with the solution, using a warm flannel. I hoped that this would knock the MRSA pathogen level back a bit, creating a space for the good bugs to gain a toehold and establish themselves.

Then I coated Rich's skin with the kefir, to try and repopulate the good bugs on his skin. When he groggily asked me what I was doing, I just said, 'Don't worry, my darling, I have it all under control.' (Which was a gross exaggeration.)

I wasn't brave enough to put my newly blended oil, or the kefir itself, directly onto Rich's wound. I couldn't face the possibility that things might go horribly wrong, and it would be all my fault. Instead, I dressed the wound with a sterile surgical dressing infused with medical honey.

## *A miraculous turnaround*

I repeated the entire procedure again that evening, and twice a day, every day, for the next week. I waited, and hoped. Rich got weaker. I milked the goats, did the shopping, got the kids to school, made soap, bottled kefir, tended the business. And prayed a lot.

And then one morning about nine days later, the angry red MRSA holes in Rich's wound seemed smaller, instead of larger. The visiting nurse and I looked at each other silently as she put the probe and the ruler away, hardly daring to hope. The next day the angry red holes seemed smaller again. And the next. Could my treatment be working?

At the end of two weeks, the MRSA holes in the wound had completely dried up and disappeared, as a puddle does when the sun comes out. The nurse took a swab from the wound itself and sent it off to the laboratory for testing. The results confirmed what we believed to be true: Rich was *completely clear of MRSA*.

I locked myself in the bathroom and sobbed hard for 10 minutes. I hadn't allowed myself to cry until that moment.

Once the infection was gone, the rest of Rich's wound healed rapidly. He was soon up and about, back on his tractor. 'Nothing wrong with me!' he said jubilantly. 'Don't know why you were making such a fuss.'

As soon as we were sure that Rich was really fully recovered, I sent my blend of essential oils – which I'd named CG Oil – off to a laboratory to have it tested. I wanted to make sure that I wasn't imagining its amazing effects.

The lab reports confirmed that our CG Oil is indeed active against MRSA, at a dilution of 0.05 percent. It also kills campylobacter, E coli, and salmonella. And it's also completely natural, safe to inhale, ingest, or apply to the skin (but only when diluted, as it's strong enough to melt plastic).

I couldn't believe how lucky we'd been. I *still* can't. I look at Rich every day and marvel that he's with us, sitting at the head of our big pine table in the farmhouse kitchen. My own personal miracle.

## How did my kefir treatment work?

Here's what I've concluded about the concoction that saved Rich's life. I believe that my combination of CG Oil and probiotic kefir performed a two-part action on his MRSA infection – it *reduced the bad bugs, and re-populated the good bugs.* The essential oils knocked back the pathogen load, enabling the beneficial bacteria in the kefir to 'take over' his skin and establish themselves.

And that's the part I believe modern medicine has been missing, all this time. Doctors are big on killing off the bad bugs with antibiotics and the like – but they don't often bother to re-populate the good ones!

### Two important lessons

Coming so close to losing a loved one was not a path I would have chosen. But I learned two important things from Rich's superbug infection, and these would revolutionize our business and change the way we thought forever:

1. Killing the bad bugs is not enough: we also have to re-populate the good bugs.

2. Kefir works on the skin as well as it does in the gut.

In 2014, a specialist from the Innovation Sector of the Welsh Assembly government came knocking on our farmhouse door. It seemed that the UK press had become aware of the story of Rich's brush with death, and his incredible recovery.

The government man listened intently as I explained what I'd discovered through treating Rich. He looked at the kefir and the CG Oil, and examined our lab results. He then set up a meeting between Chuckling Goat and Professor Jamie Newbold, head of the Institute of Biological, Environmental and Rural Sciences (IBERS) at Aberystwyth University in Wales

Professor Newbold performed extensive testing on our kefir, determining the exact genetic strains of beneficial yeasts and bacteria it contains, and finding it both safe and effective. This partnership has been very important to us, and we continue to work closely with Aberystwyth University today.

## Developing the GSS

Made bold by our discovery, we then decided to put our goat's milk kefir into the cleansers and lotions we'd been producing. Covering Rich's skin with the kefir had conquered the MRSA, but it had been inconvenient and messy. I wanted to create a kefir-based skincare product that smelled better and was easier to apply.

Getting the kefir skincare formulations right proved to be difficult and complicated, but I managed to accomplish it in the end, after many failed experiments. I applied the kefir-based cleansers and lotions to Benji's eczema, while continuing to give him the kefir to drink. His stubborn eczema completely disappeared. Another result!

Once I learned to successfully incorporate the kefir into our skincare products, our little business really took off. We won several platinum awards from Janey Lee Grace, bestselling author and natural product expert. In 2015, Hay House published my diaries of my journey to the farm and Rich's illness as *Secrets of Chuckling Goat: How a Herd of Goats Saved My Family and Created a Business that Became a Natural Health Phenomenon*. The book became a #1 Amazon bestseller.

## Kefir helps our clients

In the meantime, Chuckling Goat clients who were drinking our goat's milk kefir and using our kefir skincare were reporting tremendous results – not only with their skin issues such as eczema, but also with their asthma, allergies, hay fever, and Irritable Bowel Syndrome (IBS) all of which, as I was about to discover, are connected.

I was amazed at the intensity of the public response. **It seemed that we'd inadvertently stumbled on the answer to several intractable skin problems. One of these, eczema, has reached epidemic proportions**: in the UK alone, cases of eczema rose 42 percent between 2005 and 2009.[1] Today, the NHS estimates that one in five children in the UK suffer with eczema.[2]

People started visiting the farm, wanting to meet the goats, to ask questions, and to show us their hands, arms, and faces – free from eczema and psoriasis at long last. One man drove for seven hours to show me that he'd completely recovered from the severe psoriasis that had plagued him for 35 years.

## Listening to feedback

Working with our clients, and speaking to them on the phone about their experiences on their own healing journeys, we began to realize something:

**Drinking kefir and using kefir skincare *work together* to resolve stubborn skin conditions like eczema, psoriasis, rosacea, and acne. They heal the body from the inside and the outside.**

However, we found that putting a powerful probiotic like kefir into the body isn't a straightforward process. If there has been imbalance of the bugs inside a person's body for many years, altering the population will create a 'detox' effect.

We also found that results came better and faster when clients made some important changes to their diet. We began to offer these suggestions when people called us, asking for more information to speed their healing.

**In time, we came to call this combination of drinking kefir, applying kefir skincare, and adding gut-friendly foods to the diet, the 'Good Skin Solution' (or GSS).**

Coaching our clients through this highly individual healing process, person by person, became increasingly important to me. We took the difficult decision not to sell our kefir products through outside retailers, so we could maintain a completely personal relationship with our customers. In this way we could give them the advice they needed, and be sure that all of their questions were answered correctly.

## ✺ GSS TAKEAWAYS ✺

⊕ The Good Skin Solution (GSS) is a combination of drinking kefir, applying kefir skincare, and making key dietary changes.

⊕ The GSS is effective for eczema, psoriasis, acne, and rosacea.

⊕ Killing pathogens (disease-causing bacteria) is not enough: we also need to repopulate the good bugs on and inside our body.

⊕ Kefir works as well on the skin as it does inside the gut.

## Chapter 2

# The Good Skin Solution and You

So, let's imagine that you've come to see me in my farmhouse kitchen, as so many people have done since we started our little farm business, Chuckling Goat. Pull up a chair. I'll make you a cup of tea, and we can have a chat.

I'm guessing that you, or a member of your family, are suffering from eczema, psoriasis, acne, or rosacea, and that you've been unable to resolve it. You've probably already been to the doctor, or maybe even a hospital, where you were most likely offered topical corticosteroids, antimicrobial gels, topical retinoids, and/or antibiotics.

And while these treatments may have worked temporarily, they haven't resolved your skin problem permanently. When the medication was stopped, my guess is that the condition came rushing back with a vengeance. Maybe even worse than it was before.

## A new way of seeing your skin

You or your family member may also be suffering from food allergies, hay fever, asthma, Irritable Bowel Syndrome (IBS), fatigue, joint pain, anxiety, and depression. Does this sound about right so far? Well, don't worry – because you're not alone. I want you to know a few things.

- **Your skin condition is not your fault**. There's a huge amount of guilt and shame associated with eczema, psoriasis, acne, and rosacea because they affect the way we look, and sometimes that means we look *bad*.

- **These skin conditions have become very common** as the result of misunderstandings that we as a society have had for many years about the way things work – in our environment, inside our bodies, and on the surface of our skin.

- **Without the information you're about to read** in this book, there's absolutely no way you could have prevented your – or your family member's – skin condition **Not. Your. Fault. Okay?**

- **The Good Skin Solution (GSS) can help improve your skin**. It's going to take some time, and it will be an up-and-down rollercoaster ride, but if you're committed to the process, the chances are good that you *will* see results.

Will those results be as dramatic as my little friend Cameron's? That depends on how severe your skin condition is to begin with, how committed you are to the process, and how well you look after yourself on an ongoing basis.

What I *can* guarantee is this: the GSS *will not harm you.* It's all natural and chemical free. There are no downsides or side effects to the GSS: it won't hurt you... and it might well help. Many people also experience great additional benefits to the GSS, aside from an improvement in their skin – including improved mood, more energy, freedom from sugar cravings, and even natural weight loss.

In Cameron's case, it meant that he actually slept through the whole night for the first time in his life – and so did his mum!

## Managing your state

Living with eczema, psoriasis, acne, or rosacea, and searching for ways to resolve them, can be an emotional journey. Are you having your emotions? Or are your emotions having you? Here on the farm, we've triumphed over some pretty serious challenges by working with our mindset. We call this 'managing our state.'

We all have clear skin, good digestion, and freedom from food allergies. None of us take regular medication or use painkillers. We work hard and play hard – and have fun! We manage a big, close-knit family of 70 goats and 12 employees – all getting along together smoothly (more or less!) – as part of a high-performance business in which everything is made by hand, right here on the farm.

So when I say that something *works*, I mean it. I wouldn't be talking about it if I hadn't road-tested it under the most difficult conditions.

## Four helpful tools

Below are the four mental principles – or tools – that we use every day on the farm, in order to manage our state:

1.  **Always a challenge... never a problem**. Challenges make the world go round. Meeting challenges is how we learn, and as you'll discover in this book, meeting challenges and rising to them is how your immune system works, too.

    *Lean in* to the challenges offered in this book, and pull them toward you. Use them like your own personal gym. Face them head on. We're all stronger after we've met and risen to a challenge – just as a broken bone is stronger after it heals.

2.  **Don't be taken hostage**. In any challenging situation, there's a temptation to be taken hostage by what's going on, and simply give up. You can adopt a position of helplessness that leaves you trapped in a negative outcome. Or you can choose to fight back, and find a solution. Make choices that empower you. Keep moving forward. You are in control.

3.  **Control your focus**. Emergency responders such as police and ambulance drivers are taught to focus on where they're headed – not on the obstacles in their way. So focus on where *you* are going: not on what stands in your path. Keep your eventual – inevitable! – success firmly in your mind's eye. See your skin clear and glowing. The classic book on this topic is *You Can Heal Your Life*, by Louise Hay, the doyenne of visualization.

4.  **Ask a better question**. I learned from my lifelong friend and mentor Peter Meyers – founder of global leadership

communication company Stand & Deliver Group – that the brain works by asking questions (*I can hear you, wondering right now… Is that true? Is that right? Do I believe that? See… questions!*) Most of the time, people ask poor-quality questions. A poor-quality question is one that leaves you in a place without resources – here are some examples:

○ Why me?

○ What did I do to deserve this?

○ Why doesn't my skin ever seem to improve?

The answers to *those* questions will automatically be negative, and they'll leave you feeling stressed and depressed. There's a good reason for this: a healthy brain *leans toward the negative*. Since our caveman days, our brain been hardwired to do that – in order to protect us from danger, and to keep us alive. But when we're trying to come up with innovative solutions to existing challenges, we need to short-circuit that automatic tendency toward the negative.

## Focus on the positive

We need to ask high-quality questions that force our brain to search for a positive answer. Below are some examples of these:

• What are the most powerful things available to help me now?

• What does science know today about my skin condition that it didn't know before?

- What recent advancements might shed light on my situation?

- What can I learn today that could help me?

- How can I best help myself?

**This book will provide the answers to these particular questions.** But it's helpful to ask yourself high-quality questions like these as you move through your daily life. They will dilate your brain, and prepare you to find new solutions to the challenges you face.

## What you'll learn in this book

My purpose in writing this book is to enable you to become an expert of your own wellness. Here you will find all the tools you need to make yourself feel better. You'll get your hands on cutting-edge scientific research about the body and the skin. And as a result of learning this information, you'll no longer feel powerless.

In the following chapters, we're going to explore four things:

- **The latest scientific discoveries** about the kind of organisms we humans really are. We're at an exciting moment in medical history, as we're just beginning to discover and utilize the mighty power of something called the 'microbiome.'

- **The microbiome is the collective name for the enormous colonies of microscopic bacteria, viruses, fungi, and other living things,** both beneficial and neutral, that coexist with us, mainly in our gut, but in other places too, including our skin. These microbes have an enormous impact on our health and wellbeing.

**We're starting to understand how the microbiome works,** and why our modern **lifestyles can damage it.** We'll also take a look at how probiotics such as kefir can give the microorganisms living in our microbiome a helping hand.

- **Recently discovered facts about eczema, psoriasis, rosacea, and acne.** You'll find out what these skin conditions *really* are, and how they are **connected to the microbiome.** And you'll learn why they are so often accompanied by other symptoms such as **hay fever, food allergies, asthma, arthritis, and IBS.**

- **How adopting the Good Skin Solution (GSS)** – which is based around kefir – can make you an effective steward of your own microbiome.

## Drawing on new science

In recent years, there have been numerous scientific studies investigating the microbes that live inside our microbiome. They have revealed that these bugs have a profound influence on our health because, among other things, they regulate the response of our immune system – the body's network of organs, cells, proteins, and tissues that works together to combat illness and infection.

The findings of these studies have been published and peer-reviewed by scientists, but their implications for human health have not yet made their slow and tortuous way through the tangled labyrinth that is modern medical bureaucracy. **Most doctors simply haven't started to apply this brand-new scientific knowledge to their patients.**

I stumbled across this new science when I was searching for answers to help my family. Fortunately, my years as a newspaper reporter gave me the ability to sift through the research and find the bits that were relevant to my situation. My dedication to my family put this research ability into overdrive, and I got really lucky.

I predict that, 10 years from now, the health solutions under discussion in this book will be widely available and generally applied by doctors. But it takes a long time for Britain's NHS to trial, test, and implement new treatments.

**My family couldn't wait 10 years to resolve their medical issues, and I'm guessing you don't have 10 years to wait, either. You need answers** *now.*

So let's get started!

Chapter 3

# Heal the Gut
# to Heal the Skin

L et's begin by taking a look at how recent scientific research
has illuminated some of the root causes of eczema, psoriasis,
acne, and rosacea. In this chapter, I'll focus first on eczema,
which is the most common skin disease in the developed
world, with a huge and growing number of sufferers.[1] Later,
in Part III, we'll look at all the conditions in more detail.

## The eczema epidemic

Eczema is everywhere. Before I began this work, I had no idea
of the scale of it. Generally, sufferers don't talk about their
eczema unless they have to, and many symptoms get covered
up with sweaters and other long-sleeved clothing.

Eczema is on the increase in the UK and elsewhere in Europe,
and in the US, the National Eczema Association estimates that
a substantial proportion of the population suffers with the
condition: 31.6 million show symptoms of it.[2]

For the record, here is the *traditional* definition of eczema: 'A chronic, relapsing inflammatory skin condition... Those [affected] have skin that reacts easily to the environment and becomes flaky and itchy.'[3]

I say 'traditional,' because we're going to explore a new definition of eczema later in the book. But for now, let's see what the existing literature tells us about it:

1. Eczema, as defined by the World Allergy Organization (WAO), affects 15–20 percent of school children and 2–5 percent of adults worldwide.[4]

2. In the US, the prevalence of eczema in adults could be as high as 10 percent, which suggests that most US children with eczema continue to be affected in adulthood.[5]

3. Three percent of US adults (17.8 million people) have moderate to severe eczema requiring systemic therapy. These numbers are much higher than for psoriasis, the next most common skin complaint.[6]

4. For around 60 percent of eczema sufferers worldwide, the disorder will improve or clear up by adulthood.[7] But for those with more persistent symptoms, eczema is likely to be a lifelong illness marked by waxing and waning skin problems.[8]

5. So far, scientists have struggled to understand the origins of the condition, and there are limited treatment options available.[9]

So it's not just kids who suffer with eczema... adults struggle as well. Studies show that adults with eczema had higher out-of-pocket healthcare costs, more lost workdays, poorer overall health, more healthcare utilization, and impaired access to care compared to adults without eczema.[10]

Since eczema tends to run in families, adults with eczema not only lose sleep themselves, they are often awake during the night helping their children with the condition. If you have eczema in your family, I don't need to explain this to you – you know all about it. We received a heartbreaking letter from a mum who was in this predicament before she approached us for help.

## GSS SUCCESS STORY

*I just wanted to let you know about my little girl and her experiences with eczema. She has suffered with the terrible affliction since she was a baby (she's now six). To a large extent, I'd always been able to keep it under control: until last year, when it became out of control.*

*It was everywhere on her body, and the doctors wanted me to put her on stronger steroids. I'd tried everything else – every kind of cream, dietary changes, and remedies, and nothing had worked – so I always had to resort to steroids. These would clear up the eczema for a short period and then it would creep back.*

*My daughter has suffered teasing and bullying. Children would run away from her screaming, 'She has a disease, keep away.' We took her off all medication and tried a homeopathy route, but her skin reacted terribly. I had to keep her away from school for three weeks, and people stopped me in the street and asked if my poor daughter had 'recovered from the fire.'*

*Slowly, she became self-conscious; at the swimming pool,
children stared at her in horror, so we stopped going. One
desperate day, she looked at me and touched my skin.
'Mummy, you're so beautiful – will I ever be like you?' she
asked.*

*My despair was consolidated when a close friend who's a doctor
said that, by withholding medicine/steroids that would help my
daughter, I was being abusive. What should I do? What could
I do?*

*Then, one magical day, another mother told me about
Chuckling Goat, and suggested I research it. I did so, and gave
my daughter the Good Skin Solution. It was hard at first,
as she hated the taste of the kefir and became poorly after
suffering steroid withdrawal. But then the magic happened.*

*After three weeks on the GSS her face started to clear, and
slowly her arm, too. One beautiful day, I caught her looking
at her arms and then cuddling herself in disbelief at her skin.
She's now about to start her third course of kefir (with the
lotion, too), and is at this moment completely clear of eczema.
This is a child for whom I'd needed to get up in the night
and apply cream (at 12 a.m. and 4 a.m.), to try and keep the
eczema under control.*

*As I write this thank you note to Chuckling Goat, I have tears
running down my cheeks. You've saved my little girl. You have
no idea of the depth of my gratitude, and hers. Thank you from
the bottom of my heart.*

DR TAYLOR, CLINICAL PSYCHOLOGIST

## Your skin, your gut, and your microbiome

So you see, there *is* some good news here. Here on the farm, we've drawn on the latest science about the gut and the human microbiome to find a solution to eczema (and psoriasis, acne, and rosacea) and *it's working*. So, what have we learned that the medical profession hasn't yet started to apply to patients?

Well, as all sufferers know, topical steroids are often prescribed for eczema, because eczema *looks* like a skin condition. But in January 2015, scientific researchers made a revelatory discovery:

Eczema is not just a skin condition: it's an autoimmune disorder.[11]

It's also known that psoriasis and rosacea are autoimmune disorders,[12, 13] and acne is increasingly considered an autoimmune spectrum disorder.[14]

Autoimmune disorders sit in the gut,[15] and result from damage to the microbiome.

So logically, the simplest way to treat eczema, psoriasis, acne, and rosacea is by treating the gut itself.[16]

What does this mean for you?

You're going to have to heal your gut, in order to heal your skin condition.

### The skin is a map of the gut

Once you get your head around this concept – and this book aims to help you do that – you'll understand why creams alone have not worked to help your eczema, psoriasis, acne, or rosacea. It's because these skin conditions are all just *symptoms* of a deeper gut disorder.

At Chuckling Goat, what we discovered as our clients took their courses of kefir, applied our kefir skincare, and reported the results back to us, was this: *our skin is really just a map of our gut.* Heal the gut, and eczema, psoriasis, acne, and rosacea will diminish. It takes time – but they will improve!

This might seem like a strange idea at first. **But scientists now know that** *our gut is directly connected to our skin.* For example, studies have shown that children with eczema have different bacteria in their gut to those kids who don't have eczema.[17]

And in fact, your body is doing you a favor. You can't see what's going on inside your gut, and so it's easy to ignore it. But when your gut paints a map on your skin, in the form of eczema, psoriasis, acne, or rosacea, it's time to wake up and get concerned.

Consider it your body's warning system. You've been given a visible signal that something's wrong – and a chance to resolve the problem.

So join me know as we take a trip into the depths of the gut – home of the incredible microbiome – and learn how the life inside it affects our skin....

## ✺ GSS TAKEAWAYS ✺

✦ Eczema is the most common skin condition in the industrialized world.

✦ New research shows that eczema is not just a skin condition – it's an autoimmune disorder. Acne, psoriasis, and rosacea are also autoimmune disorders.

✦ The bacteria in our gut play a role in autoimmune skin disorders.

✦ In order to heal your skin, you must heal your gut.

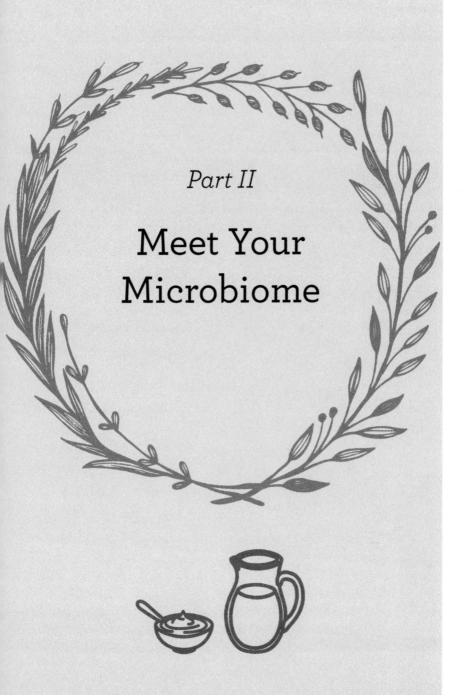

*Part II*

# Meet Your Microbiome

Chapter 4

# You Are a Superorganism!

The human gut is a dark and mysterious place – hard for us to see, and even more difficult to understand. But scientific research has now revealed that sitting inside our intestines is a vast and complex community of microscopic organisms that has evolved alongside us to help us perform the basic functions of life.

This internal ecosystem is called the microbiome. It's located largely in our gut, but our skin, our genitals, our mouths, and our eyes also have microbial colonies. (We'll explore the skin microbiome in Chapter 7.)

In the gut, the microbiome consists of 2kg (4.4lbs) of microbes – mainly bacteria, but other microbial species, too – all living and thriving in a complex, cooperative web.

## The microbiome

Some of the bacteria in the gut microbiome are simply along for a free ride; these are known as 'commensal' bacteria, and we'll be looking more closely at them later on. Others, called symbiotic bacteria, work with us in a mutually beneficial relationship. And of course, lurking in the background are the pathogens: nasty opportunistic microbes that sometimes cause disease.

So what determines whether the pathogens in our microbiome co-exist peacefully with us, or break out and cause a problem? That's determined by the overall makeup and balance of our microbiome. Nothing exists in isolation; it's a question of how individual bacteria relate to the entire system.

It's only recently, through the groundbreaking work of the Human Microbiome Project, that we've come to understand how mind-bogglingly extensive this internal ecosystem is. Less than 10 years ago, scientists had only discovered 200 species of bacteria as cohabitants of our bodies.

**Today, it's estimated that more than 10,000 different microbial species occupy the human microbiome, and more are being identified all the time.**

## The jungle in your belly

Inside your gut microbiome are up to a quadrillion/septillion ($10^{24}$) bacteria, all doing their thing right this very minute: contributing to digestion, producing vitamins, and promoting gastrointestinal health.[1] Just to help you visualize that quantity: this is the same number of stars found in our observable universe.

**These microbes form real living communities, just like the ones you see in nature programs on TV. They live side-by-side,**

competing for nutrients, overthrowing one another, or even benefitting from each other.

Scientists at Oxford University in the UK have found that inside the gut microbiome, there are prey and predator species battling with each other all the time.[2] Awed researchers look up from their microscopes to report that 'Competition among bacteria is brutal and fierce.'[3]

The inside of the gut resembles a jungle, and in fact, that's the easiest way to understand it. Imagine that your gut is the gorgeous Amazon rain forest: full of complicated life forms such as lizards, leaves, frogs, flowers, fish, jaguar, and deer – all competing, eating, breeding, fighting, and going about their day-to-day business.

Except in the case of your gut bacteria, the day-to-day business is you! It's their job to break down your food and turn it into building blocks for skin cells, muscle cells, organ and bone cells, and so on. They also protect you from pathogens (those disease-causing microbes) and maintain your immune system.

**You are the planet – and your bugs are the busy, productive little inhabitants of that planet. Without them, you couldn't survive for even one second. Sterilize your gut, and you die.**

Strange as it may sound, your entire body is actually a 'superorganism,' made up of different kinds of bacteria. The number of bacterial cells living within the body of the average healthy adult is estimated to outnumber human cells by 10 to one.[4] Let me say that again:

**You have 10 times more bacterial cells than human cells!**

*You are really just a constellation of bacteria* – a big walking, talking 'bacterial mat.' Researchers in this field even describe we humans as 'hosts,' and say that our job is to help maintain natural stability in the gut by acting as 'ecosystem engineers.'

## We're all holobionts

This realization that we're all 'bacterial mats' is such an important and powerful shift in the way that we think about ourselves, that scientists have come up with a nifty new word to describe it. The word is 'holobiont,' which means 'a host organism (plant or animal) in interaction with all associated microorganisms.'

To understand this concept more clearly, imagine that you're an iceberg. The human, or 'host,' bit of you is the tiny tip that sits above the water. The rest of you is under water; nine out of 10 of your cells are tiny bacterial 'symbionts,' meaning 'an organism living in symbiosis with another.' The whole of the iceberg is called the 'holobiont.'

**So, 10 percent human host + 90 percent bacterial symbionts = 1 holobiont.**

### *You're not just human!*

Cool, eh? All this time, we've been thinking of ourselves as individuals, but with this new understanding, we can see that was a *massive* oversimplification. The pronoun 'I' is just *so* yesterday – there's no such thing as 'I': you're actually a 'we'!

We humans are biomolecular networks consisting of visible hosts, plus millions of invisible bacteria. These bacteria have a significant effect on how we develop, which diseases we catch, how we behave, what we choose to eat, and possibly even our social interactions and our choice of mate.[5] The whole is much greater than the sum of its parts.

Does this matter? Yes, it does. For one thing, it alters everything we know about our immune system. Holobionts have an advantage over an individual organism: they have more ways to respond to threats. This is probably why humans are holobionts to begin with: it gives us a great edge in survival.

For example, if a holobiont is attacked by a pathogen that the host cannot defend against, another symbiont may step up and fulfill the job by manufacturing a toxin that can kill the invader.

## Interrupting the 'conversation'

Looked at in this way, the bacteria in your microbiome are as much a part of your immune system as your own immune genes. In fact, scientists are now beginning to understand the immune system as a 'conversation' between us and the critters living inside our bodies. In a healthy person, the microbes in the gut stimulate the immune system, and the immune system responds.[6]

Like whales singing to one another in the ocean, our human cells 'talk' to our bacterial cells, and that conversation makes up our immune system response. It's beautiful, mysterious, and – here's the main point – ultimately fragile and easily interrupted.

In much the same way that we've interrupted whale song by making the oceans so noisy that those creatures are unable to communicate, navigate, or hunt properly, we've loaded our microbiome with DNA-altering chemicals, toxins, and antibiotics that have interrupted the delicate back-and-forth exchange of our immune system. And the result for our skin has been disastrous.

## GSS SUCCESS STORY

*I just thought you might like to know how kefir has improved my son Steffan's psoriasis. We've both been taking kefir for six months, and the improvement is very noticeable in him. We seriously believe in this product as, after 35 years of going back and forth to doctors/hospitals, nothing has ever come close to relieving this condition.*

*You won't believe how happy I am to have found something that's helped my son's condition improve – in just six months!! Seeing him like he was, really got me down, but this has truly restored my faith in the fact that there are natural products out there that really do work.*

*For as long as I live, I will never again take a doctor's pill for psoriasis.*

EMYR ROBERTS

(See photographs in the colour section.)

## ❧ GSS TAKEAWAYS ❧

⊕ Inside your gut is the 'microbiome': 2kg (4.4lb) of bacteria and other microbes.

⊕ Your microbiome is a complex ecosystem full of living organisms.

⊕ You are a superorganism called a 'holobiont' – made up of 10 percent human cells and 90 percent bacteria.

⊕ Your immune system is a 'conversation' between your human cells and your bacterial cells.

Chapter 5

# Getting to Know Your Good Bugs

Now that you understand you're part of a holobiont, you need to learn a little bit more about the other helpful life forms – the symbionts – with which you share your body. We can't hope to be good stewards of our internal ecosystem without good information. So here are a few key things about the bacteria living inside your microbiome.

1. They're not passive – they're interacting with you!

2. Sometimes they want different things than you do.

3. In order to get their way, they release toxins and endorphins into your system.

All those tiny bugs inside your microbiome aren't just sitting back and relaxing. Instead, they're active participants in a two-way engagement with you.

# Your gut is manipulating you

You control the mouth of the superorganism, and when you eat, you make the weather for all the little critters inside you. But a recent study has shown that, rather than just passively living off whatever nutrients we send their way, our gut bacteria influence our food choices in order to make us eat the things that *they want*.

Different bacterial species need different nutrients; some prefer sugar, and others live off fat. But they not only fight with one another for food, and to retain a foothold in the ecosystem. **Your bugs often want different things than you do, and they're not shy about going after their goals.**

Your gut bugs have the ability to impact your behavior and mood by altering the neural signals in your vagus nerve. They change taste receptors and produce toxins to make you feel bad when you don't eat the things they want, or release chemical rewards to make you feel good when you *do*.[1]

So the bacteria inside your gut are actually manipulating you. It's important to understand this, because it's what makes it so hard to change your diet: the bugs inside you are playing you like a big marionette, trying to force you to give them what they crave. It's a carrot and stick approach.

## GSS SUCCESS STORY

*Hi. I've just ordered my third lot of kefir after having used your lotions since the beginning of the year. Thank goodness my lovely husband read about your products in a Sunday newspaper supplement, as I was suffering with an undiagnosed skin condition – perhaps eczema – that made me look ancient. Previously, I'd never had a skin problem in my life!*

*I was prescribed steroids and lots of antibiotics, but nothing worked. The skin on my face and hands was terrible and very painful. No one in the medical profession had an idea what was causing it. I ordered your lotion and my skin became much better.*

*I then tried the goat's milk kefir. It's an acquired taste, but I'm now actually hooked on it and have never looked back. My dermatologist can't believe it! It has been a miracle. I never thought I would look like my normal self again, so big thanks to you and the goats!!!*

SUE JEPSON

## *They are what you eat*

Animal studies have shown that 20 minutes after a meal, gut microbes produce proteins that can suppress food intake.[2] If you think in terms of evolution, it's not too difficult to see how this came about. Mealtimes bring a mother lode of nutrients to the bacteria inside the gut. In response, they divide to replace any members they're about to lose in the development of waste products.

Since gut microbes depend on us for a place to live, it's to their advantage that their population remains stable. So it makes sense that they have a way to communicate to the host when they're not full, nudging us to ingest more nutrients – or stopping the process when their population is stable.

Fortunately, this relationship is a two-way street. **We can affect the population balance of the bugs in our gut by changing what we eat...** as long as we can withstand their nasty little attacks while we do it!

And once we've done the hard work and swung the balance in favor of the bugs that live off healthy things, they will help us by craving and rewarding our consumption of those things, instead of the sugary nasties. Firm but fair, right?

Our food choices have a huge impact on the microbiome in our gut. It's a whole ecosystem, and it's evolving on a timescale of minutes.[3] The microbes are so small, and have such short lifespans, we can alter their population fairly quickly, simply by changing our diet and introducing specific bacterial species through taking kefir. These are the central planks of the Good Skin Solution (GSS).

## Meet your commensal bacteria

So, now that we know a bit more about the crazy, magical universe we have living inside our gut, we can see how delicate it is and how complex. Next, I'd like you to meet some old friends who have lived right alongside – and inside – you, all the time...

Here's another nifty new term for you: *commensal gut bacteria*. Scientists use this to describe all the non-harmful bugs living in and on the body. 'Commensal' is a lovely word – in its early English use it meant 'eating from the same table,' but in the late 19th century, biologists started using it to mean 'Living in a relationship in which one organism derives food or other benefits from another organism without hurting or helping it.' Since that time, the scientific sense has almost completely overtaken the original use of the word.

So if you have severe eczema, and your GP is trying to convince you to use immune suppressants to treat it, you can casually toss in the following phrase next time you see her: 'Before we go down that route, I'd like to try out some oral and topical immunotherapy first, to boost the activity of the commensal bacteria in my immune system.' (Do let me know what she says!)

## We are the bugs, and they are us

Anyhow, when you see the word 'commensal,' in an article about the human gut, it's a good sign that you're reading about the work of scientists who are working with the updated concept of the entire holobiont. If you want to get really specific about it, symbionts are bacteria that help us, and commensals are neutral bacteria that are just along for the ride.

We happily co-exist with all the teeming symbiotic and commensal bacteria inside us, despite the fact that they share many similar features with the infectious bacteria against which our immune system reacts.[4] Yet, if you ate a dodgy piece of chicken that had just a few tiny Salmonella cells on it, your immune system would immediately react with a powerful inflammatory response.[5]

So how does our immune system decide which bacteria to attack? In all the legions of bacteria inside us, how do we pick out our targets? Answer? We don't. *They* do.

Strange as it may seem, these critically important decisions are made not by our own human immune cells, but by the non-human bacteria that live inside us. Since we are their home, they hold the key to our immune system. They then 'enforce' their decision by hijacking the cells of the immune system.[6]

*We are them, and they are us.* For the practical purposes of discussion, there's not an awful lot of difference between the 'human' part of your immune system, and the 'commensal' part. We've been so intimately connected to our bugs, for such a long time, that at this point, there's just no teasing us apart.

**So, it's time to reboot our concept of 'self.' Our commensal bacteria have evolved to look and act like us. They live inside us for our entire lives. They are *part* of us.**

As far as our immune system goes, we cannot make a distinction between 'human' cells and 'bacterial' cells. They are constantly cooperating, in one big dance.[7]

## GSS SUCCESS STORY

*I just wanted to say that your kefir lotions and cleansers have been a life-changer for my three year old. She has had severe eczema since birth, and while we've been able to maintain the skin on her torso, arms, and legs, her face never clears up – despite the use of various steroid creams (which have thinned her skin so much).*

*Now we use the Sensitive range daily, and the Break-Out range if she has a flare-up. Her skin is now amazing. We are so grateful to you.*

CAROL-ANN MAYBERRY

# The 'right' kind of dirt

This is a pretty big shift in the way that we see ourselves. When you're dealing with autoimmune challenges like eczema, psoriasis, acne, and rosacea, as well as food allergies, hay fever, and asthma, you don't have to do it alone... because for you, there's no such thing as alone!

**You are a holobiont. That means you're always right at home with a trillion of your closest bacterial buddies.**

But when you lose touch with those buddies, then things start to go wrong. Back in 1989, British epidemiology professor David Strachan suggested that a lack of childhood exposure to harmful germs and fewer childhood infections are to blame for the sharp rise in allergies. This idea became known as the hygiene hypothesis.[8]

Twenty years or so on, it turns out that this line of thinking was close, but not exactly right. Apparently the problem is not that we're *too clean* – so you don't need to stop cleaning your house, or start trying to expose yourself and your children to dangerous pathogens. Studies show that routine daily or weekly cleanliness habits don't really reduce the levels, or alter the types, of microbes in our home environment.

**Try as we might, we can't create a truly sterile environment in our homes, any more than we can on our skin.**

## *Step away from the idea of sterile*

As fast as we remove microbes by cleaning, they are replaced, via dust and air from the outdoor environment, or from microbes that are constantly being shed from our bodies, and from pets, food, and other items brought into our homes.[9]

So, forget about trying to make yourself or your home sterile. It's just not going to happen. And anyway, it was never the real problem. The underlying idea that you need to be exposed to microbes to regulate the immune system is correct. But according to recent research, it's simply not the case that children who have fewer infections because they live in more hygienic homes, are more likely to develop asthma and allergies.[10]

So, if hygiene isn't the problem, then what is? Well, it turns out that we're missing out on the *right kind of dirt*.

**What's the right kind of dirt? It's stuff that contains the right kind of bugs.**

I'm not talking about the infectious nasties that cause respiratory infections such as colds, influenza, and measles, and gastrointestinal infections like campylobacter poisoning and norovirus, but *the good bugs with which we co-evolved*.[11]

## Get dirty!

The best way to reconnect with the 'right kind of bugs' is to get back out into the environment in which we first met them, back when we were co-evolving with them – the great outdoors.

So head outside and get some dirt on your skin. Play with your pets. Walk on the beach, take off your shoes and get your toes into the sand. Pick strawberries or blackberries. Go for a muddy walk. Take the kids to visit a farm. Have a stroll in the woods.

Nature is packed full of the microbes you need to get your immune system back to its best. And since you're going to have to work with your good bugs in order to help your skin condition, in the next chapter we'll be looking at one of the things that harms them the most – antibiotics.

## ✿ GSS TAKEAWAYS ✿

- ✛ The bugs in your system engage in an active, manipulative relationship with you.

- ✛ They reward you if you eat what they need to feed on, and punish you if you don't.

- ✛ The term for the good bugs inside you is 'commensal bacteria.'

- ✛ Your commensal bacteria make the decision about which other bacteria to attack as pathogens.

- ✛ It's important to get back in touch with 'the right kind of dirt,' which contains 'the right kind of bugs.'

## Chapter 6

# Antibiotics and the Microbiome

So, now that you know you're a superorganism, and that trillions of microscopic bugs call you home and support your health, you may like to consider this fact: taking antibiotics (for your skin condition or for any other health issue) is like pouring bleach into a river.

**Antibiotics not only kill the bacteria that are causing your infection, they destroy everything else in the gut microbiome as well.**

Although antibiotics are powerful and effective drugs for treating bacterial infections – and they can be lifesavers in certain situations – these days they are increasingly being prescribed when they're not needed.

Antibiotics are completely ineffective, for example, against fungal infections or viruses. Recent studies show that currently, as much as 50 percent of all antibiotic use is inappropriate.[1] And because of this overuse, antibiotics are becoming less effective over time, leading to a rise in antibiotic-resistant infections.

## A vicious circle

The misuse and overuse of antibiotics – and topical corticosteroids, too – can create harmful 'iatrogenic' conditions. Now there's a two-dollar word for you! An iatrogenic condition is one caused by a medication that's supposed to make you better. Increasingly, it seems that our most common go-to drug solutions – antibiotics and steroids – are causing as many problems as they're solving.

Antibiotics can become a 'subtraction stew' solution, which means the more you use them, the worse you become. Antibiotics lay waste to the microbiome, which harms the immune system, leaving us more susceptible to infection.

So we get sick again, return to the doctor for more antibiotics, which further damage the microbiome... and so on.[2] And scientific research published in 2016 showed that exposure to antibiotics early in childhood is related to an increased risk of both eczema and hay fever in adulthood.[3]

**The real problem lies in the fact that the harm done by antibiotics to the microbiome is rarely fixed. The gut is just left in a damaged condition, and over time, this can lead to increasingly serious secondary infections.**

Topical corticosteroids, too, which are intended to help skin conditions such as eczema and psoriasis, can actually *cause* more intense problems over time. Steroids are applied to the skin but because the underlying autoimmune issue, which sits in the gut, remains untouched, they don't work. So we go back and ask for stronger steroids. We then overuse those in a bid to get some relief... and into another vicious circle.[4]

## The outdated 'germ theory'

So what's going on here? Why is the medical establishment handing out solutions that only make things worse? Fundamentally, the problem is that modern medicine is based on a concept of disease called the 'germ theory.' Researched and developed by French chemist Louis Pasteur in the 1860s, the germ theory was adopted by later scientists, gradually gaining acceptance in Europe and the US.

Basically, the germ theory states that the human body is *sterile*, and that problems begin when 'germs' (microorganisms) invade the body and cause disease.

The germ theory led, ultimately, to the development of more hygienic medical practices and to the introduction of the first antibiotic, penicillin, in 1941, which revolutionized the treatment of bacterial infections. In the decades since then, we have continued to call the body's microorganisms 'germs,' and have waged constant war against them, using antibiotics as our point-and-shoot weapons.

What's wrong with this? A lot. Pasteur was a smart guy who did a lot of amazing things, but he was working in the 19th century, using the optical lenses of the day. He simply couldn't *see* then, what scientists can see now. He didn't *know* what microbiologists know today. And what can we see? What do we know now, that Pasteur didn't?

## *You are not a blank slate*

For one thing, the research by the Human Microbiome Project shows us that there's *nothing sterile* about the human body. In fact, you are the furthest thing from sterile that can be imagined. You are the planet, remember? You are the Amazon rain forest. You are a living ecosystem, not a sterile environment.

And what happens when you pour bleach into the Amazon River? Or introduce antibiotics into your own living microbiome? Sure, the antibiotics will kill what's causing the infection. But they will destroy the good bugs in the microbiome as well. Your inner ecosystem will be knocked out of balance.[5] And you'll pay the price for years to come because you are not a blank slate.

**Your system is not sterile: your microbiome is a living, changing, adjusting, interactive system.**

Put simply, the 'germ theory' is outdated science. And a medical system based on it will inevitably have problems, because many of its solutions are based on a concept that's obsolete. We know better now.

As author and teacher Stephen Harrod Buhner says in his book *Herbal Antivirals: Natural Remedies for Emerging and Resistant Viral Infections*, 'Bacteria and viruses are not a "virulent other."

'They are, instead, intimately interwoven into the underpinnings of life on this planet. They cannot be killed off without killing off every form of life on Earth. This is the great error of the 19th/early-20th-century view of nature that continues to plague us.'[6]

*Remember: we are the bugs – and they are us!*

You are a holobiont. And 'germ' is just an old-fashioned – and insulting – word for microbial life. *There's no such thing as a germ* – only holobionts, symbionts, and pathogens, all swirling and competing and cooperating in a vast ecosystem.

### GSS SUCCESS STORY

*I found the Calm-Down kefir lotion lovely and soft; it absorbed well into the skin and the smell was light and relaxing. It most definitely did the job and calmed down my red, angry, hot and itchy skin. I used it twice a day for approximately a week and my flare-up died down completely.*

*I want to say thank you for all your products: the Break-Out cleanser and lotion and the drinking kefir are really helping my daughter's acne as well. She is on her third round, and every day her skin is looking a little clearer. It took some convincing to get her to take the kefir in the beginning, but now she can see the improvement herself, it's the first thing she drinks in the morning, without question.*

*Thanks so much to you and the goats.*

CAROLINE CALVERT

## The danger of antibiotic resistance

Look, this is not just some interesting intellectual exercise. The outdated germ theory, and the stubbornness of our medical system in clinging to it, is now officially putting all our lives at risk.

Because *antibiotics are just not working anymore.*

I hope you never have the terrifying experience I did: staring blankly at a doctor as he explains that he's very sorry, but your loved one has a life-threatening infection. And there's absolutely nothing he can do to help, because that infection is now resistant to all antibiotics.

But that day is looming for all of us, faster than you may think. Rich and I may have been among the first to experience that nightmare, but we won't be the last. We were just the initial canaries in the coalmine – the early warning signs of a bigger problem, yet to come.

You've probably read the headlines, and you've no doubt heard the worrying news stories. Sure, you understand that there are increasing numbers of resistant bacteria out there that no longer respond to antibiotics. But you tell yourself: *Surely someone will do something to save us? All those smart men in their white coats will solve the problem.*

## The end of the antibiotics road

Well, I'm here to tell you that (for the time being, anyway) they are *not*. It takes 15 years to develop a new antibiotic, and there are currently none in the pipeline. No one is coming to save us. Don't believe me? Ask former British Prime Minister David Cameron.

While he was in office (May 2010–July 2016), Cameron commissioned an independent review to look into the growing threat of resistance to antibiotics, and *why no truly new class of antibiotics has been introduced for more than 25 years.*

'This is not some distant threat but something happening right now,' Cameron said. 'If we fail to act, we are looking at an almost unthinkable scenario where antibiotics no longer work and we are cast back into the dark ages of medicine where treatable infections and injuries will kill once again.'[7]

Here's what that review revealed:

- **Antibiotic-resistant diseases** could cause an extra **10 million deaths globally** every year, unless urgent action is taken.

- **Superbugs,** currently responsible for 700,000 deaths a year, **could kill more people than cancer** by 2050, at a cost to the global economy of £63 trillion.[8]

The fact is, we've reached the end of the antibiotics road. We need to come up with something new. We're going to have to save ourselves... holobionts, symbionts, and all. We need to ask some better questions.

We need to become good stewards of our internal ecosystems – not point-and-shoot destroyers. It's all about balance, about interacting with the critters inside us – and restoring health and balance in our microbiome.

## Are you overusing antibiotics?

We all take antibiotics – and we take them a lot. It's estimated that 40 percent of all adults and 70 percent of all children take one or more course of antibiotics every year, and billions of food animals are given them, too.[9]

Now, don't get me wrong, there are many times when antibiotics are necessary and lifesaving, and we should all give thanks for that!

**But we often take antibiotics when they are neither necessary nor lifesaving.**

When you or your child are ill, it's so tempting to ask your doctor for antibiotics, or to take the prescription handed to you without asking any questions. You may reason that taking antibiotics can't hurt, and it might help. You might know that they carry the risk of side effects, but perhaps you reckon that risk is small.

The problem is, some doctors prescribe antibiotics for respiratory tract infections, such as coughs and colds, that would clear up on their own.[10] Studies show that half of the estimated 100 million antibiotic prescriptions each year for respiratory tract infections may be unnecessary.[11]

The majority of people who see their doctors for a sore throat or acute bronchitis are prescribed antibiotics, but only a small percentage of those people actually need them. Those illnesses are usually caused by viruses, and antibiotics (which, remember, only treat bacterial infections) don't help.[12]

## Harming, not helping

Were you aware that *antibiotics harm you the minute you start taking them*? Antibiotic use has been linked with a host of health issues, including digestive dysfunction, diarrhea, ulcerative colitis, obesity, problems with food absorption, depression, immune function, sepsis, allergies, and asthma.[13] They can also cause tendonitis, inner-ear problems and hearing loss, impaired kidney function, and other problems.[14]

But why does this happen? It's because antibiotics don't just kill the bad bugs that are causing your infection. They kill *many good bugs inside your microbiome as well.* Remember that lovely Amazon rain forest – full of living things like tiny flowers and tall trees, birds and deer and jaguars? Well, taking antibiotics is like *firebombing that rain forest.* Total wipeout of every living thing.

If you've ever suffered diarrhea or IBS after a course of antibiotics, you've experienced this effect for yourself, first hand. The good bugs have been destroyed, and can no longer do their important jobs of digesting your food and running all the systems in your body. And unless you re-seed them, those good bugs won't *ever* grow back – not properly.

Your gut works in much the same way as your garden. If you clear a space with antibiotics and leave it empty, it *will* fill up – but not with beautiful flowers. That space will become filled with tough, fast-growing, opportunistic pathogens: the 'weeds' of the gut.

Researchers have also discovered that the long-term effect of antibiotics is even worse than was feared. Antibiotics also kill intestinal epithelium.[15] This is another nifty new word for you: epithelium – the stuff that lines blood vessels and organs throughout the body. Your glands are made of epithelial tissue.

Epithelium is found in the walls of your capillaries, the lining of your lungs, the ducts of your kidneys, pancreas, and salivary glands, and in the lining of your intestines. So if you're killing intestinal epithelium with antibiotics, you're *drilling holes* in the essential parts of your body where you absorb nutrients and store your immune system. Not ideal, really, is it?

## Secondary infections

Have you ever noticed that once you start taking antibiotics, you get more infections, rather than fewer? It seems contradictory, but it's true: taking antibiotics over a long period of time can lead to severe secondary bacterial infections.

It turns out that the good bugs in your gut keep your immune system primed to effectively fight infection from invading bad guys. When you kill off the good bugs with antibiotics, the immune system is no longer primed.

You can think of this as like starting a car: it's much easier to get it moving if it's idling, than if the engine is cold. In the same way, if your immune system is already warmed up, it can cope more readily with the pathogenic (bad) invaders.

Normally, your neutrophils (white blood cells) are constantly being primed by bacterial signals, so they're warmed up and ready to go if a nasty microbe invades the body. They are sort of 'idling' and the baseline system is already turned on. But when you take broad-spectrum antibiotics, you turn that system off. The system is 'de-primed' and will be less efficient at responding quickly to new infections.[16]

Prolonged use of antibiotics throttles down your immune system, so it no longer runs at peak efficiency. But there is good news:

The use of probiotics – like kefir – can undo the damage caused by antibiotics.

It's been shown that keeping your immune system 'primed' by eating foods enhanced with such 'friendly' bacteria may help counteract the negative effects of antibiotics.[17]

## Be aware of the risks

Here's the really important thing for you to know: the danger of antibiotic overuse isn't just about the creation of a hypothetical superbug that might attack some stranger. Antibiotics begin to damage your microbiome the instant you begin to take them. Studies have found that many people don't understand those risks,[18] but the risks are immediate, and very real.

So don't just close your eyes and turn over your family's health to the doctor. Become an intelligent consumer of health services.

You need to take responsibility, and do some independent thinking – for yourself, or on behalf of your family member. If your doctor offers to prescribe an antibiotic, ask if it's absolutely essential; ask whether it will *really* help your condition.

And *always* follow a course of antibiotics with a course of kefir, for at least nine weeks.

## ✸ GSS TAKEAWAYS ✸

⊕ Antibiotics that are prescribed to treat pathogenic (disease-causing) bacteria also have a devastating impact on the good bugs in our microbiome.

⊕ Modern medicine is based on an outdated concept of disease called the 'germ theory'. This holds that the body is sterile, but we now know this is far from the case.

⊕ The growing problem of resistant bacteria created by antibiotic overuse means that we're all increasingly at risk.

⊕ Doctors commonly overprescribe antibiotics when they *will not help*.

⊕ Antibiotics start harming us the minute we take them.

⊕ Antibiotics increase our risk of a secondary-infection spiral.

## Chapter 7

# The Gut–Skin Connection

You may be wondering how all this information about gut bacteria, the immune system, and antibiotics relates to your eczema, psoriasis, rosacea, or acne. After all, these conditions affect your *skin*, right? Well, as researchers in the US have recently discovered, our immune system – 80 percent of which is found in the gut – has a direct influence on our skin.[1]

And, just as you were getting used to the idea of trillions of bugs living inside your gut, you now need to know that you also have trillions of bugs living on your skin, too! This collection of critters is called the 'skin biome.'

## Introducing your skin biome

The skin biome was a 'hot topic' at the 23rd World Congress of Dermatology in 2015. Until recently, a key dermatological concept was that the skin was a barrier designed to keep things out, rather than interact with the environment.

But recent advances in skin biology reveal that the skin is a dynamic organ, packed with beneficial organisms that can benefit us – if we let them do their job.

We need to keep the wellbeing of these organisms in mind, when we do things that affect the skin.

One of the most important ideas that came out of the Human Microbiome Project was that nearly everyone carries 'bad bug' pathogens in the gut. But in healthy individuals, pathogens don't cause disease: they just co-exist happily with their host and the rest of the microbiome. It's only when the entire system falls out of balance that those bad bugs begin to act up and cause problems.

This is also true on the skin biome. Wiping out the good bugs that live there – by using 'antibacterial' products, for example – leaves empty spaces for the pathogens to proliferate and turn nasty. Antibacterial products disrupt the delicate balance between good and bad bugs and knock the immune system out of kilter, which increases the risk of allergies, especially in children.[2]

## More bugs = better skin

Both the gut and the skin form part of the immune system. In fact, the immune system exists wherever there's potential for the body to be harmed by coming into contact with the outside world. As the body's largest organ, the skin represents a major site of interaction with the microbes in our environment. The skin and the gut are two of the primary locations where we need protection, and they are intimately connected.

Your skin biome is partly governed by an evolutionarily ancient branch of the immune system called 'complement.' The clever complement system works like a molecular alarm and first responder, leading the counterattack against 'microbial insult' when the bad bugs try to break in. It also has anti-inflammatory functions, and may be responsible for maintaining a diverse set of microbes on your skin, keeping it healthy.[3]

It might seem strange to focus on the fact that your skin is teeming with invisible bugs. But do bear in mind that most of these are *good* bugs – helpful, commensal, non-pathogenic bacteria. They perform critical services for us: mainly blocking the bad bugs from getting too strong a foothold.

Scientists have found that the bacteria that normally live on our skin actually protect it from infection. Our skin health relies on commensal cells interacting with our immune cells.[4] This means that your immune system, your gut, and your skin are inextricably linked, and must all function together to keep your skin in good shape.

**When it comes to your skin condition, the main idea is to repopulate the bugs inside your gut *and* those on your skin. Result? Healthy, glowing skin.**

The more types of bugs you have on your skin, the merrier! Fewer bugs means more skin issues.

## Thrown out of balance

It's becoming increasingly evident that many skin diseases are caused not by bad bacteria, but by 'dysbiosis' – an imbalance in the microbial community. Once again, it's knocking out the entire ecosystem that causes the problems on your skin.

We're too quick to try to pin the blame on 'bad microbes,' or 'germs,' which we then try to kill. Point-and-shoot has always been our default solution, and it's time for that to change – in our dealings with the microbiome as well as the outside world! It's time to consider 're-balancing,' instead of 'killing off.' We need to think about how we can nurture our microbes rather than eradicate them. They evolved with us for a reason.[5]

We want to keep our skin biome enriched and healthy, thriving with lots of different kinds of healthy bugs – just like our gut biome.

### GSS SUCCESS STORY

*I haven't used my prescribed creams and steroids for my eczema for a while now. Instead, I've just been using your Break-Out lotion. Apart from my wrist, which has always been hard to control, my hands are practically eczema free. Just some small scars, but these are barely noticeable.*

*I'm happy because in the past, my hands have been red raw and it was distressing.*

GILLIAN COLLINS

# What harms the microbiome?

Like any natural ecosystem, your gut and skin biomes are fragile, and vulnerable to attack. Antibiotics can cause great harm to your good bugs; we discussed this earlier. Here are some of the other things that can damage them.

## Sugar

When everything's working well inside your microbiome, it's a win-win situation. The good bugs produce energy and vitamins, and help keep the bad bugs under control so they can't harm you. In exchange, you (as their polite host) help maintain their habitat and provide them with an environment that helps them grow.

However, a problem arises when you eat sugar. Sugar feeds the bad bugs – like pathogenic E. coli. Remember that pathogens are inside you all the time – it's when they get out of control that things go wrong.

**When your diet is low in fiber and high in sugar, the bad bugs go crazy! Essentially, you're feeding the wrong side – the enemy.**

The bad bugs, strengthened by the sugar, become bold and start stealing iron from your own host cells. Your body responds by ramping up immune activity, basically starting a little microbial war. Result? Obesity, diabetes, and inflammation-related disorders such as eczema, psoriasis, rosacea, and acne.[6]

## Stress

To be a smart holobiont, you must understand a key point: diversity is good. It's true in the outside ecosystems of the planet, and it's equally true inside your body. The more diverse your microbiome, the better your health. This is why probiotics like kefir are so helpful for your gut and skin.

A landmark study, published in January 2016, showed that squirrels with lower levels of stress hormones also had more diverse microbiomes. When their stress levels went up, their bug diversity went down, and levels of potentially harmful bacteria increased.

**So, more stress = less diversity = more bad bugs.**

This study was the first demonstration of its kind to be conducted in a natural environment, and the first to show that there's a link between stress and microbiome diversity in the wild.

Researchers concluded that 'Bacterial diversity within animals and people is emerging as an essential component of health, and this study provides data that shows the link between low stress and a healthy microbiome.'[7]

## Antibacterial products

According to new research, an antimicrobial and antifungal agent called triclosan, which is found in many consumer products, can rapidly disrupt bacterial communities found in the gut. Triclosan was first used as a hospital scrub in the 1970s and is now one of the most common antimicrobial agents in the world.

It's an ingredient in shampoos, deodorants, toothpaste, mouthwashes, kitchen utensils, cutting boards, toys, bedding, socks, and trash bags. It continues to be used in medical settings, and can be easily absorbed through the skin.[8]

Triclosan has been linked to cancer and bone malformations in animals.[9] It's in a class of environmental toxicants called endocrine-disrupting compounds (EDCs), which are thought to negatively impact human health by mimicking or affecting hormones.[10] There is growing concern among the scientific community and consumer groups that EDCs are dangerous to humans at lower levels than previously thought.

What does this mean for you and your skin condition? In a nutshell, it means microbiome damage and allergies.

**If you have eczema, food allergies, hay fever, or asthma, exposure to triclosan may be making it worse.**[11]

## Is your microbiome damaged?

How can you tell if you or a family member have microbiome damage? Imagine microbiome damage as a tree with many leaves. These leaves manifest as different conditions in different parts of the body. They may *look* like separate issues, but they all stem from the microbiome-damage tree. And the trunk of the tree sits in your gut.

- **On the skin**, microbiome damage can appear as **eczema, psoriasis, rosacea, or acne**.[12]

- **In the joints**, it can show up as **rheumatoid arthritis**.[13]

- Inside the gut, it can appear as **food allergies**[14] and **IBS.**[15]

- In the nervous system, it can show up as **chronic fatigue**[16] or **nerve pain.**[17]

- In the lungs, it can appear as **asthma.**[18]

- In the nose and eyes, it can show up as **hay fever** or **seasonal allergies.**[19]

- In the brain's behavioral center, it can appear as **anxiety and depression.**[20]

If you present with any of these symptoms, your doctor may diagnose three or four different conditions – and prescribe painkillers, antibiotics, or steroid creams, none of which will really help. As you now know, these just damage the microbiome further, making the problem worse.

Modern medicine tends to break things apart, and look at each problem in isolation. But nature doesn't work in isolation, and neither does your body. All of these issues are connected to microbiome damage. Resolve the damage to your gut, and these symptoms will improve over time. We've seen it and heard it from our clients, time after time. It really is that simple!

## Becoming biome-friendly

Of course, we all want to create a safe, clean, and hygienic environment for ourselves and our families. But as we learned earlier, our definition of 'clean' has gotten off-track, and we've developed the erroneous notion that:

1.  It's possible to sterilize everything around us (it isn't!) *and*

2.  Sterile is good. (It's not.)

All we're doing with our misguided attempts to kill off all those nasty 'germs,' in our guts and on our skin, is wiping out good bugs and leaving the space open for nature's weeds to jump into the vacuum. So, how can we act intelligently and cooperate with the vast soup of tiny microbial life that exists all around and inside us?

First of all, if you use antibacterial liquid soap that contains triclosan, I want you to walk straight over to the bin and throw it away! Check your toothpaste while you're at it; same actions apply. (Not all toothpaste brands display the product ingredients on the tube, so you may need to Google yours to find out what's in it.) In fact, in order to protect your microbiome, you should avoid using *any* products containing triclosan.

And stop using antibacterial soaps and hand washes altogether. Here why…

## Finding the right kind of clean

Healthy skin – or a healthy gut – is a space grab. It's all about good bacteria and bad bacteria, fighting it out for a toehold. The question is – who's going to win? The answer: whichever side you support with your actions.

The reason for the rise in allergies and chronic inflammatory diseases such as eczema is that we've been pursuing *the wrong kind of clean*. Let's say it one more time for the record: *you are never going to be sterile*. When it comes to the human body, there's no such thing as sterile. You are *made* of bacteria. You can never kill them all – you would be destroying your own components.

So any product whose label features the word 'germs' (remember, that's a derogatory term for microbes) and promises to kill 99 percent of them, is offering the wrong kind of clean.

**The wrong kind of clean kills off most of the bugs, and leaves a largely empty space behind for the serious nasties to occupy.**

This is a *really bad* idea. Because in nature – and remember, we *are* a part of nature! – when a space is cleared, it will be filled. But what with? Opportunists. The toughest, fastest-growing things that can get in there, and take over the space that you have so considerately cleared for them. Bad bugs.

Some of those bad bugs are already there, right on site. That product may promise to kill 99 percent of them, but the few that survive are, by definition, the really strong ones – the so-called 'persistents' that were able to outlast the attack.

By using antibacterial products, we kill off the bad bugs' weaker competitors, leaving lots of room for the bad bugs to breed and repopulate.

## Getting clean with probiotics

So, if calling the body's microbes 'germs' and getting rid of most of them is the wrong kind of clean (and creates horrors like MRSA), then what is the *right* kind of clean?

How about probiotic cleansers that preemptively fill up the empty space with good bugs? That's an idea proposed by Professor Mark Spigelman of the University College London (LCL) Centre for Infectious Diseases and International Health.

Spigelman says the time has come to re-evaluate the concept of using antibiotics, and scrubbing hands and wounds with antiseptic soaps. He suggests that saturating the skin with 'good' bacteria may offer us better protection against deadly germs.[21]

Spigelman is now calling for a study to be set up in hospital units in which antibiotics would be banned; this would allow us to explore alternative health protection measures against MRSA. He says: 'Perhaps we should be thinking about using probiotics, even dipping our hands after thorough washing into a solution that contains harmless bacteria, which could then colonize our skin and prevent pathogenic bacteria from settling on it.'[22]

*Preemptive probiotics offer the right kind of clean.* Any student who has grown bacteria in a laboratory knows that bacteria don't grow on top of each other. Here's the bit we've been missing all this time, with our antibacterial soaps and antibiotics.... After you clear a space, you've got to put the right kind of bugs in, to fill up that space. Otherwise the bad bugs will settle there and beat you to it.

**Making a dent in the bad bugs is only the first part of the job. To finish it off, you also have to *fill that space with good bugs.* That's the right kind of clean.**

## Restoring bug diversity

There's an increasing chorus of agreement with this theory among scientists. 'Healthy microbiota may be a way to address growing problems with antibiotic resistance,' says Andrey Morgun, from the Oregon State University College of Pharmacy in the US. 'Instead of trying to kill the "bad" bacteria causing an illness, a healthy and functioning microbiota may be able to outcompete the unwanted microbes and improve immune function.'[23]

What we need here is some harmony. We need to do something to restore balance to our internal ecosystem, which has been knocked out of whack by all the chemicals and other nasties we've been dousing it with. We need to restore the diversity of our gut and skin microbiomes.

This is where the GSS comes in:

**Drinking kefir, applying kefir-based skincare and eating to support the microbiome will bring you back into harmonious balance with all the invisible friendly critters that surround you, inside and out!**

You'll find out how to put the GSS to work for you in Part IV of the book.

## ✤ GSS TAKEAWAYS ✤

✤ The trillions of bugs living on the surface of your skin are called the 'skin biome.'

✤ Both your skin and gut biomes can be damaged by antibiotics, sugar, stress, and antimicrobial skincare products.

✤ Microbiome damage can appear as eczema, psoriasis, acne, rosacea, chronic fatigue syndrome, anxiety, depression, IBS, food allergies, hay fever, and asthma.

✤ Triclosan, a chemical compound commonly found in antibacterial soap and toothpaste, and many other household products, harms the microbiome.

✤ Healthy skin is a space grab. You need to support and enhance the presence of good bugs on your skin and inside your gut, to crowd out the bad bugs. The best way to do this is by using probiotic skincare.

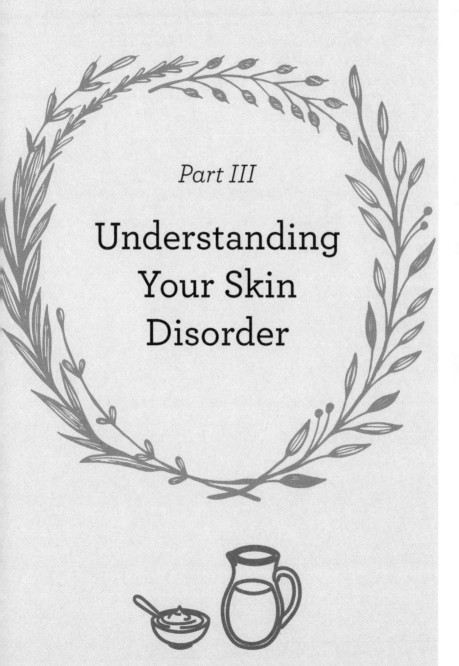

*Part III*

# Understanding Your Skin Disorder

## Chapter 8

# Eczema and Allergic Disease

We've seen why a well-functioning gut and skin microbiome (and in turn, immune system) – chock full of beneficial bacteria – is so essential to our health and wellbeing. Now we're going to take a look at how damage to the immune system can cause chronic, inflammatory skin conditions like eczema, psoriasis, acne, and rosacea.

Let's start with eczema. Remember the statistics we talked about earlier? Roughly 20 percent of children in the industrialized world suffer from eczema. But that number drops to around 5 percent of the adult population.

Many people say, with some relief, 'Well, I had eczema as a child, but I grew out of it.' Unfortunately, it's not that simple. Eczema rarely rides alone. The truth is, eczema is frequently just the first stage of something more complicated, called *allergic disease*.

## Are you on the allergic march?

After their eczema symptoms have disappeared, many people find that they move on to the next stage of allergic disease: food allergies. Then comes hay fever, followed by asthma. If this progression sounds familiar to you, then you may be on what's known as the 'allergic march.'

There's a typical 'allergic career' for many people with allergic disease, and it generally follows this pattern:

1. Eczema in infancy
2. Food allergies in childhood
3. Hay fever, then
4. Asthma during the 40s.[1]

Based on recent science, I'd like to propose a fifth member to this ugly little cabal: Irritable Bowel Syndrome (IBS). A study by Rush University Medical Center in the US found that patients with allergy symptoms (hay fever and allergic eczema) reported a high incidence of IBS.[2]

So, a typical allergic career may progress in this way:

1. Eczema
2. Food allergies
3. Hay fever
4. Asthma
5. IBS

If you have eczema, you may also have some or all of these other allergic conditions. And if you do, again, you're not alone! In Europe, one in four children suffer from allergy,[3] and as much as one-third of the entire population is affected,[4] making allergic disease the 'non-infectious epidemic' of the 21st century.[5]

Some estimates suggest that in the US, nearly 4 million days of missed work each year are due to allergy symptoms.[6]

The incidence of allergic disease is high and escalating. Allergic diseases such as asthma and hay fever are problematic for about 30 percent of the population in the industrialized world. Researchers have developed various treatments to control allergy, but so far doctors haven't been able to cure it.[7]

**Here's the thing about the allergic march – if you allow it to proceed, it will just trundle through its progressively nasty stages.**

To get an idea of the severity of this problem, up to one-third of US children with eczema may also have a documented food allergy.[8]

A study conducted in Melbourne, Australia, found that children who had eczema, particularly when it occurred with hay fever, were nine times more likely to develop allergic asthma in their 40s.[9] And US studies have shown that between 50 and 70 percent of children with severe eczema will go on to develop asthma. By comparison, in the general population, only 9 percent of children and 7 percent of adults have asthma.[10]

## Stopping the allergic march

But here's the amazingly good news – the allergic march can be halted! Studies show that the rigorous treatment of childhood eczema and hay fever can prevent the development of asthma in adulthood.[11]

No matter where you are on the allergic march, it *can* be stopped. And if it is stopped, it won't progress onto its next stage. Catch it early, at the eczema stage, and your child will never progress to having asthma in his or her 40s.

That's one of the great successes of the GSS – halting the allergic march.

In view of this new information, I'd like to propose (for the purposes of discussion) an updated definition of eczema: 'An autoimmune disorder which often represents the first stage of allergic disease, producing symptoms of reddened, itchy skin, and frequently progressing to food allergies, hay fever, asthma, and IBS.

### GSS SUCCESS STORY

*I've always had allergies, mainly to dairy products. As a baby, once I went onto formula milk, I was covered in eczema; my mother still describes my skin as having been as scaly as a snake's!*

*Fast-forward 28 years, and I'd been taken off wheat by a herbalist to aid my severe hay fever. I wasn't always as strict with my diet as I should have been, but nine months ago, I stopped eating food with wheat, dairy, and added sugar, as the eczema on my hands was worsening – I had patches of it on my neck sometimes too.*

*I had a particularly bad six months. There was a lot of change, and I was so miserable in my job, it was making me anxious. As a result, my eczema started to spiral out of control.*

*I would wake in the night with my hands feeling as if they were on fire. They had blisters, which would then burst and turn to open wounds. My hands were so sore, I was scared to wash them, and I couldn't wear my rings because my fingers were so swollen. (Of course, none of the steroid creams I tried worked, and I know now why, thanks to Shann's excellent website and information.)*

*I tried a number of alternative therapies over this time – including homeopathy and Chinese herbs – but nothing really worked. There was a small improvement but nothing major, and the herbs especially took a lot of time effort, and expense.*

*I then became very unwell. It began with some sort of infection, which progressed to full-on pneumonia. I was off work for a month, and my system was pumped full of antibiotics for three weeks. During this time my hands actually improved, but as soon as I stopped the antibiotics they were worse than ever.*

*So I decided to Google raw and organic goat's milk or cream and came across Chuckling Goat. When I read the website it was literally as if all my dreams had come true! Although I didn't want to get my hopes up in case it didn't work.*

*The kefir arrived, along with the Break-Out lotion and cleanser. I didn't take to the taste of the kefir, but I just knocked it back, telling myself it was medicine. Within three days my hands were no longer hot at night and I was sleeping through as a result – which felt amazing.*

*Within seven days the blisters weren't coming up daily, or hardly at all actually. Within 12 days the wounds on my hands had pretty much healed! I was totally amazed, as was my boyfriend – he's a farmer and very 'traditional!'*

*My neck also completely cleared and my hands are now a million times better than they were! I'm so grateful for the GSS – without being too dramatic, it has changed my life. I'm on my third course of drinking kefir. My hay fever is 70 percent better this year, and I put that down to no wheat and dairy and the kefir! It's miracle stuff!*

GEORGIE HULBURD

(See photographs in the colour section.)

## The body's first line of defense

So, why does the allergic march affect the skin (eczema), gut (food allergies and IBS), sinuses (hay fever), and lungs (asthma)? The answer is that all of these locations are *barrier sites* where your insides meet the outside world. These are the places where, logically enough, your immune system is concentrated, in order to protect you against external attack.

Barrier sites – the skin, gut, sinuses, and lungs – limit the inner body's exposure to allergens, pollutants, viruses, bacteria, and parasites. Understanding how your immune system works in these places will help you see how and why the allergic march occurs.[12]

**Like a fence designed to stop intruders, your skin acts as a barrier, protecting your body from the hundreds of irritants with which you come into contact daily.**

## Skin barrier breaches

Scientists have found that healthy skin has strong and secure tight junctions (cell-to-cell connections), which act like a gate controlling the passage of water and particles.[13]

In the skin of eczema patients, however, these same junctions are loose and porous. So if you have eczema, your skin barrier is *leaky*, allowing intruders such as dust mites, pet dander, pollen, mold and others, to slip through the holes in the barrier. This in turn sets off the alarm inside your immune system, causing havoc throughout all the other barrier sites.[14]

Barrier problems like these 'tight junction defects' (places where the lining of the intestine and airways is weakened) are also a common feature of other inflammatory diseases, such as asthma and IBS.[15]

**What eczema, asthma, and IBS have in common is that the connective tissues involved – skin, airways lining, intestine lining – are loose and porous, thus allowing intruders to enter.**

The body responds with an inflammation reaction – and this is what causes the eczema in the skin, asthma in the lungs, and IBS in the gut. Probiotics like kefir are useful in these cases because they reduce inflammation, and help seal up the leaky tissues.

## ❧ GSS TAKEAWAYS ❧

⊕ Eczema is often just the first stage of the 'allergic march.'

⊕ The allergic march commonly proceeds through the stages of eczema, food allergies, hay fever, asthma, and IBS.

⊕ The lungs, sinuses, gut, and skin are affected by the allergic march because all these places are barrier sites, where the immune system meets the outside world.

## Chapter 9

# Adventures Inside Your Immune System

So, we've talked about the relentless progression of the allergic march: from eczema, to food allergies, to hay fever and asthma.... But how does the allergic march actually get started? What kicks it off?

Well, it turns out that the villain of the piece is something that's produced by our own immune system – immunoglobulin E (IgE) antibodies. An antibody is the immune system's 'weapon': a protective protein that's produced when foreign substances called 'antigens' invade the body.

IgE antibodies are commonly found in the body's barriers sites – the lungs, skin, and mucous membranes. IgE is a powerful immune system weapon, designed to protect us from parasitic infections.

But too much IgE in the body is commonly associated with severe allergic reactions.

In order to understand more clearly what your IgE antibodies do, and how your barrier sites work, let's turn to the best teacher of all – your own body.

## Your life as a B cell: boot camp

Imagine that I've waved a magic wand, shrunk you down to microscopic size, and inserted you inside your own immune system. Here we go:

*You are a young, naive, inexperienced B cell – one of the two main types of lymphocytes (white blood cells) that play a vitally important role in the immune system. You're due to become an infection fighter – a pretty cool job in the bacterial world.*

*On your first day, you nervously report for training. You sit down in the classroom with the other novice B cells. Suddenly the door opens and a big, tough T cell walks in. You all shiver with fear.*

*'Who are you?' asks the T cell softly, looking around the room.*

*'We're the new B cells,' says a cell behind you, timidly.*

*'I can't hear you, soldiers,' bellows the T cell. 'Who are you? And call me sir!'*

*'We're B cells, sir!' everyone shouts.*

*'That's better,' says the T cell. 'And who am I?'*

*Long silence.*

*Finally, the T cell says: 'I'm your mummy.'*

*One of the cells behind you laughs. The T cell takes off his mirror shades and stares down at him for a long moment.*

*'You think that's funny?' he asks.*

*The B cell who laughed swallows hard before answering: 'No, sir.'*

*'Too right, it's not funny. It's the truth. I'm a regulatory T cell – Treg for short. And what I regulate – is you! While you're here in training, I'm your mother, father, and nursemaid. I tell you who you are, and make you into what you're going to be. And if you go rogue, I'm here to put you down like a rabid dog. Do you understand me?'*

*Frightened silence.*

*'I said, do you understand me?'*

*'Yes, sir!' all the cells shout in unison.*

## Immune system training

*Treg puts his shades back on and leans back against the desk, folding his arms.*

*'That's better. Now, who's ready to start learning how to fight infection?'*

*All the hands go up. 'Right, so who knows where we are?'*

*Silence.*

*Treg sighs, and pinches the bridge of his nose. 'Let's take this very slowly. What kind of cells are you?' he asks.*

'Lymphocytes, sir?' you venture cautiously.

Treg nods, and you feel yourself glow.

'That's right. And so lymphocytes start out in the...'

'Bone marrow?' you offer.

'Excellent! Right now, we're in the bone marrow of the host, and we'll remain here until your training is complete. After that, you'll all migrate to the spleen, where you'll be activated. Inside the spleen, you'll be differentiated into your final classes, and then – and only then – will you be considered mature B cells.

'You've got a long road ahead of you, and until you're activated, you'll take no action of any kind, without my permission. Everyone understand?'

Everyone nods nervously.

'Now, we are part of the immune system. Anyone know which part?'

Silence.

Treg sighs again. 'Okay, the immune system has two parts – the innate and the acquired. B cells like you – and T cells like me – are part of the acquired immune system: the learned or "memory" bit. You are part of the host's memory section of the immune system.

'You'll learn to recognize each different kind of bacteria, fungus, or virus that you meet. And the next time that particular bug tries to invade the body, you'll be ready for it and able to fight it off more easily. That's why the host will only catch some infectious diseases – like measles or chicken pox – once.'

*Treg shudders before continuing: 'And goodness knows, we don't want a repeat of chicken pox! Horrible. So that's why you need to pay attention, here in training. You'll gain knowledge and experience of invaders over time. We hope.'*

*He grins around the room. 'Oh, lighten up, little B cells. You're going to be just fine. Any questions?'*

*'Sir, will we have any weapons to fight with?' a cell at the back asks nervously.*

*'Your antibodies are your weapons,' Treg replies. 'You'll be instructed carefully in how to use your antibodies. They are dangerous weapons. If misused, they can harm the host. And if the host goes down, we all go down.'*

*'Where are our antibodies, sir? Do we get assigned them?' a B cell asks.*

*Treg laughs out loud. 'You've been carrying them with you all along, little B cell! Look down at your DNA,' he says.*

*Everyone looks.*

*'See that thing in your middle with five Y-shapes radiating out from a center point? That's your own personal antibody. The double-sided end is the bit that you connect to the invader, to zap it. The handle is the bit that sticks to you. Got it?'*

*'Yes, sir!' The B cells shout, staring down with fascination at their own DNA.*

## Choose your weapon!

*Treg then turns out the lights and fires up a Powerpoint presentation.*

*'Now then, let's talk about the different classes of antibodies you may end up carrying. They're also known as immunoglobulins, or Ig for short. Which type of Ig, or antibody weapon, you end up with is determined by where in the host you're called to patrol, and what threats you'll face there.'*

*Treg clicks to the first slide – it's captioned 'IgM.' The slide shows a center point with five double Y-shaped rays radiating from it, like a throwing star.*

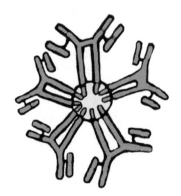

IgM (Immunoglobulin M): the first antibody
produced by the body to fight infection

*'IgM is for beginners,' Treg continues. 'Everyone starts out with IgM – that's what you have right now.'*

*You look down at yourself again. He's right.*

*'You'll note that IgM has five legs. Some of you will carry on forever with IgM, and never change. And there's nothing wrong with that!*

*Perfectly good antibody. Lot of need for it. If you end up carrying IgM, you'll be working mostly in the bloodstream.'*

*He clicks again for a new slide; this one says IgA.*

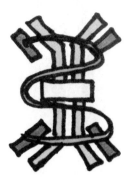

IgA (Immunoglobulin A): found in high concentrations
in the body's mucous membranes

*'This is IgA. Notice that it's simpler than big and clunky IgM – more specific, easier to handle. We've trimmed off three legs here, just left a Y-shape at either end. IgA is mostly found on mucosal surfaces, like those in the throat and intestines.*

*'Hosts with low IgA are at higher risk for developing recurrent infections and autoimmune disorders – so I'll expect all of you who end up carrying IgA to do your work well!'*

*He glares at the B cells, who shrink back.*

*'Those of you carrying IgA will be working mostly in the lungs, digestive tract, and body's secretions: saliva, sweat, tears. IgA is specific for allergies. Your job will be to help keep mucosal bacteria in check. And then –Treg pauses dramatically – there's IgE.'*

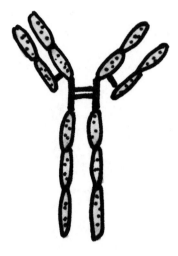

IgE (Immunoglobulin E): the rarest and most effective antibody

*'Ooooh,' all the cells say, as the slide appears. IgE looks silvery, streamlined: somehow shinier and more deadly looking than any of the immunoglobulins that came before it.*

*'Cool,' says the B cell behind you, laughing. He jabs his neighbor in the ribs and says: 'That's what we want to end up with, right?' His friend looks impressed.*

## Playing with fire

*'IgE is the ultimate weapon,' Treg continues.*

*'You only need a pinch. It's incredibly strong, designed to fight intestinal worms and other parasites. It's the rarest and most effective antibody. Even tiny traces of IgE can trigger extremely violent allergic reactions in the host.'*

*He looks around the room, at each B cell in turn, before saying: 'If you play with IgE, you play the end game. IgE is a kamikaze weapon. Anyone know why?'*

*The laughing B cell behind you jabs his mate in the ribs again: 'Boom!' he says.*

*Treg walks over to him slowly and stares down. Laughing B cell and his friend both visibly shrink in their seats.*

*'You are correct. Deploy IgE, and after a few brief moments, I will come and end your life – to ensure that you don't continue to spray IgE into the host.*

*'Your life will be short, but glorious. We call this apoptosis – cell death. And that's my job – to keep you from going rogue. A rogue B cell spraying IgE will cause a massive allergic attack inside the host. Do you all understand?'*

*Treg snaps the lights on again. All the cells sit very still.*

*'Please, sir, how do we choose a weapon?' the laughing B cell asks. You notice that he's no longer laughing.*

*'Right now, you're all carrying IgM,' Treg says. 'When you face an invader, you'll switch your own weapon class by changing to the appropriate antibody. When that time comes, you will know. That's what this training is for.'*

*'How do we switch weapon class, sir?' a cell calls out.*

*'You will cut your own DNA,' Treg replies, soberly.*

*'Can we change back?' the cell asks.*

*'No. As you might have guessed by looking at the picture, once you cut up your IgM, it's abolished. You can't go back.'*

*'What if we cut it wrong?'*

*'Don't cut it wrong.'*

*'But what if we do?'*

*'Well, son, we call that cancer.'*

## Your life as a B cell: barrier patrol

*Fast forward. So now you've completed your B-cell training and are out on patrol in the skin barrier. It's your first day on the job, and you're feeling pretty good about yourself. You pat yourself down as you stroll along, checking for all your equipment.*

*Your IgM antibody weapon, stuck to the front of your DNA, ready to alter as needed and shoot at any invaders? Check. A big slobbery, tail-wagging macrophage (a pathogen-eater) walking on a leash next to you, ready to attack and gobble any attacking foreign bodies? Check.*

*And last but not least, your hand-grenade-style canister of TSLP (thymic stromal lymphopoietin) – a notification molecule that enables you to communicate with your fellow B cells if something goes wrong. Check.*

*At the first sign of any disruption or intrusion, you've been trained to pull the pin on that TSLP canister. It will immediately boil like purple smoke through the corridors of the host, alerting your B cell colleagues in the host's other barrier sites – the sinuses, lungs, and gut.*

## Sounding the alarm

*Suddenly, up ahead, you see an invader. What is it? It's huge. It's a birch pollen molecule! One of the worst allergens possible. It's 10 times your size and the ugliest monster you've ever seen.*

*How did it get in? Clearly, the host's skin has not been producing enough good fats to keep it healthy and hydrated. Dry skin means chinks in the barrier, and itching. Itching means scratching, which means that foreign molecules can be physically driven deeper through the skin barrier. And that means...*

*'Barrier breach!' you shout, as loudly as you can. 'Skin barrier breach! Itch alert! Invasion!'*

*You rip your TSLP canister off your belt, pull the pin and detonate it. Purple smoke starts to billow out of it in choking waves, spreading rapidly down the passages to alert your fellow B cells, up in the sinuses.*

*Once they get the alarm, they will start to pour out loads of mucous, ready to flush out any invaders. Clouds of TSLP are also spreading rapidly to alert the B cells in the lungs, who will start to constrict the airways, to prevent invaders from gaining access.*

*In the gut, your other B cell classmates will begin to create muscular ripples and watery fluid, ready to repel the invader.*

*You snap the leash off your macrophage, releasing it. 'Go get it, boy!' you cry, and the macrophage runs forward growling, launching itself straight at the invader. You watch helplessly as the birch pollen molecule, big as a train, bats the macrophage out of the way. The macrophage whimpers, twitches once, and then lies still.*

*This is bad, you realize. This is serious. It's time for the big guns.*

*You take a deep breath, and look down at the antibody you're carrying. Right now you're still carrying five-pointed IgM antibody, like all your classmates. But IgM is not going to work on this monster. You think back to what your trainer Treg taught you.*

*IgE? You shudder. No, IgE isn't necessary for a birch pollen molecule, thank goodness. Too extreme, too dangerous.*

*IgA? That's the one – good for allergies, and birch pollen is an allergen. IgA is strong enough, but not too strong. You take a deep breath, hold your cutter firmly and slice deeply into your own DNA: three cuts, just as you were taught, turning the five-legged star of IgM into the two-legged shape of IgA. You pull it out, and stare at it: it looks just like the slide you saw in immune class. You feel a glow of triumph.*

## Conquering the invader

*Boosted by your success so far, you vault toward the birch pollen and stick both of the Y-ends of your DNA onto it, trying to get full contact. Its cell membrane is slippery, and you slide along the surface. It bats at you, but fortunately misses.*

*It's howling like a hurricane now, and you can't get a good lock on it. You try again. This time you leap onto its neck, riding it like a bull, and clamp your antibody down on it again. You make the connection – just in time. You click the latch, lock in, and start to spray IgA straight into the invader.*

*It's working. You clamp your knees onto the birch pollen molecule and spray the IgA into it with all your strength. The monster is thrashing wildly and howling, but it seems to be slowing down. It's starting to wrinkle and shrivel. It collapses to the ground, and you jump off, twirling your IgA molecule over your head triumphantly. You've done it – success!*

Is this science fiction? No, in the main, everything above is correct. (Although I admit to embellishing a few details – for example, macrophages do eat infectious agents, but I have no proof that B cells actually walk them on leashes!)

## The link between eczema and asthma

Scientists once believed that food allergies cause eczema. Now they think that it's the other way around – eczema comes *first*, and actually causes food allergies, which then progress to hay fever and asthma: the rest of the allergic march.

In 2009, research uncovered what could be the key to the allergic march. It showed that a substance secreted by damaged skin circulated through the body and triggered asthmatic symptoms in allergen-exposed laboratory mice.[1]

These findings suggest the problem of the allergic march starts with damaged or defective skin. A tiny fault in our genetic code that results in the skin not producing enough good fats, or 'bio-lipids,' to keep skin healthy and hydrated.

This leads to dry skin, which fails to keep the skin barrier intact. So the skin barrier – which as you now know plays a critical role in protecting us from allergens in our environment – breaks down and fails to do its protective job.[2]

## The TSLP 'alarm'

The B cells in the damaged skin sense this problem, and send out a cry for help. They do this by secreting a cytokine (signal molecule) called TSLP (thymic stromal lymphopoietin), a compound capable of provoking a powerful immune response.

Cytokines are the means by which cells communicate with each other – we can think of them as the 'walkie talkies' of the immune system (as in the birch pollen invasion scenario I've described above).

**Remember, the skin is the first of the body's barrier organs, so an invasion at the skin level is a major fail for the immune system.**

Because the B cells in the skin are so effective in secreting TSLP into the circulatory system, the substance travels throughout the body.[3] This 'TSLP alarm' lets all the other barrier sites know that the walls have been breached, and invaders are at the gates.

Research found that when the TSLP reached the lungs of the laboratory mice, it triggered the hypersensitivity that we recognize as asthma in humans.[4]

TSLP also makes you *itch*. Itching leads to scratching, and scratching causes skin injury; the damaged skin then releases more TSLP… which leads to more itching, more scratching, and so on. It's a vicious circle – and you're caught right in the middle of it.[5]

Another of TSLP's functions is to *increase inflammation* – because that's the way the immune system deals with problems. For us, inflammation means the production of watery liquid in the eyes, mucous in the sinuses, watery fluid in the bowels – all of which are the body's attempt to flood out, shut down, or block out invaders from penetrating deeper into the system.

So, fundamentally, too much TSLP in your system means you'll have an allergic inflammation in your lungs, skin, and gut.[6]

## The key to allergy

In 2010, studies on human cells conclusively showed that TSLP specifically directs immune cells to produce an allergic response, proving that it's central in the development of allergic diseases like eczema, food allergy, and asthma in humans.[7] And all because your poor hard-working B cells are trying to communicate with one another, to protect you from invasion!

Under normal circumstances, TSLP serves as an alarm to call in the immune system to heal breaches in the body's barrier organs. Healing turns the alarm off and sets everything back to normal.

But if damage in the skin barrier stems from a genetic abnormality, the skin *can't* return to normal. And, like a car alarm that just keeps wailing and driving everyone mad, the constant stream of TSLP into the system triggers the ongoing disaster of the allergic march.[8]

**The presence of TSLP has now been definitely linked with asthma, as well as eczema.** The epithelial cells lining the airways in the lungs of asthma patients are continually producing TSLP – just like that car alarm that can't be shut off.[9]

## When B cells go rogue

We're going to learn more about that alarm – and look at how using probiotics can shut it off. But first, let's head back into your immune system to see what happens when things go *really* wrong....

*As you stand over the shrunken body of the birch pollen molecule you've just destroyed, you heave a deep sigh of relief. Victory. You shove your newly deployed IgA weapon back into its holster.*

*But as you look around, you hear the sound of more fighting. B cells are pouring into the area and purple clouds of TSLP are boiling everywhere, being sucked quickly down the hallways of the veins to alert the sinuses, lungs, and gut.*

*You see larger breaches in the skin barrier. There are gaps everywhere, and through them, monstrous invaders are piling in – more pollen molecules. But wait, what's that over there? Is it... a dust mite? You've heard stories about them, but you've never actually seen one. It's three stories high, hairy, and armored like a tank. You feel sick, just looking at it. How will you ever fight such a thing?*

*Then, from behind you, you hear a howl. Something comes rushing past you. You're knocked to the side. Looking up, a little dazed, you recognize Laughing Cell from your training class – the one who was so enchanted with IgE. His friend is right behind him, and they are both charging toward the monstrous dust mite.*

*'IgE, IgE!' they chant.*

*Simultaneously, they stop, yank out their IgM immunoglobulins, and start hacking at their own DNA. They cut off one, two, three legs... 'Noooo!' you shout. You try to stop them, but it's too late. They've both made that last critical cut.*

## The power of IgE

*They're now both wielding IgE weapons – icy, dangerous, green, and glittering like razors. Somehow both B cells look different, too – pale and filled with menace. They advance on the dust mite, one from each side, and slice into it, easily. You recall from class that IgE is designed for worms and parasites, so the dust mite is no match for it.*

*Unable to look away, you watch the B cells finish off the dust mite. But the light of battle is still in their faces. Eyes bulging, they're still shouting 'IgE!' and swinging around, trying to find something else to kill.*

*'Are you okay, soldier?' you hear someone say.*

*You look up, and there's Treg. You're so relieved to see him that you nearly burst into tears. He'll fix everything. He'll stop those rogue B cells. That's his job.*

*He jerks you to your feet, and looks down briefly at your weapon. 'IgA, I see! Well done. Get back in there – we need every cell. This is a serious pollen attack.'*

*Then his eyes fix on Laughing Cell and his buddy, running around like lunatics, waving their IgE weapons, slicing chunks out of everything within sight.*

*He groans. 'I always knew it would be those two.'*

*He tightens the belt on his own weapon and starts running after the two B cells, who are now swelling up, looking monstrously large.*

*'Stop right there! Put the IgE down, and step away!' Treg commands them. Gibbering and frothing from the mouth, the two B cells advance on him from either side.*

*'This is your last warning, B cells,' Treg shouts. 'Put it down, or you'll leave me no choice!'*

*Maddened, the two B cells rush in on him. Treg swings his own weapon at Laughing Cell's buddy. It connects, and the B cell crumples into a heap. But Laughing Cell sinks the long, icy blade of his own IgE into Treg's side, and hurtles off into a side vein, screaming crazily at the top of his lungs and slashing at everything in his path.*

*You run over to Treg, who is kneeling over the body of the dead B cell, holding his side. He looks up. His face is grey.*

*'Sir,' you say. 'You're hurt! Can I help you?'*

*He shakes his head. 'You can't help me, soldier. And if there's not another T cell around to stop that rogue B cell from spraying IgE everywhere, no one can help any of us. This is an eczema attack for sure.'*

### Summing up IgE antibodies

So what has our adventure inside the immune system taught us so far?

IgE antibodies are a particular type of powerful antibody normally used to protect against parasites. In Western lifestyle countries, where parasites are less frequent, high levels of IgE are frequently associated with allergic disorders.

In people with a genetic predisposition, the immune system overreacts and begins to produce IgE antibodies against harmless things like pollen, dust mites, or animal hair. Certain cells then work with IgE to attack the allergens. This process can cause symptoms of allergy such as hay fever, eczema, and asthma.[10]

Basically, the idea here is that IgE is a misused weapon of protection. It's a good immunoglobulin, designed to fight parasites and worms, that goes wrong.

But the news here isn't all gloomy, as there may be a hidden upside to your eczema. Because IgE is so powerful, it also kills tumor cells, and may prevent cancer! Numerous in-depth studies have shown that people with raised levels of IgE, commonly found in eczema patients, may be at a lower risk of developing certain types of brain and skin cancer.[11, 12]

Can you see now how complex and delicate your immune system is? Your interior universe is an ingenious, dramatically balanced place, with many trillions of constantly moving parts. Some of these living inhabitants actually function by mutating, altering their own DNA, and then hovering close by to kill one another if the process goes wrong.

## Kefir to the rescue

So with this picture firmly in our minds, let's reconsider our use of antibiotics and immunosuppressant drugs that some doctors seem to think are such a good idea for eczema and psoriasis.

Essentially, in order to prevent a B cell from going rogue and spraying IgE everywhere, these drugs firebomb the entire immune system. The complex and intricate system that's trying to protect you is simply wiped out of existence. It's like burning down the entire Amazon rain forest just to get rid of the mosquitoes.

**But, as we discovered on the farm, if the immune system isn't functioning properly, there *is* an alternative to shutting the whole thing down with immunosuppressants. That alternative is kefir, the powerful probiotic that helped save my husband's life.**

You'll discover more about kefir in the next part of the book, but for an illustration of how it works inside the immune system, let's head back in there one last time.

When you last saw him, Treg had been overcome by the rogue B cell spraying IgE, and things were looking bleak.

## A vision in white

*You lean over Treg, helplessly watching him fight for breath. Things are looking very bad now – the holes in the skin barrier are getting wider, and pollen, dust mites, and animal hair molecules are pouring through. Your fellow B cells are valiantly fighting the monsters, but many of them are going down.*

*Choking purple clouds of TSLP are everywhere and in the distance, you can hear Laughing Cell still screaming maniacally as he capers on, spraying IgE all around the host. It's a disaster.*

*Suddenly, you hear a strange sound. You look up. Marching around the corner is an entire platoon of unfamiliar soldiers. They're dressed all in white – gleaming like new tooth enamel, so bright that you have to shield your eyes. You gasp.*

*Treg opens his eyes. 'What is it?' he croaks.*

*'I don't know,' you say. 'I've never seen anything like them before.' You prop Treg up gently, so he can see.*

*'Kefir,' he says, marvelling. 'The host has taken kefir. The probiotics are here.'*

*Suddenly, abruptly, the new white-coated soldiers are everywhere. They're at the skin barrier, sealing up the holes in the wall. They're speedily overwhelming the dust mites, pulling them over and kicking them aside. They're moving through the B cells, passing out extra IgA molecules for use against the allergens. The tide of the battle is turning so rapidly, you can hardly believe it.*

*Three of the white-coated soldiers jog over to where you're holding Treg. They gently move you aside and get to work on the wounded Treg, bandaging him and jabbing him full of things that you can't see. In a minute he's back on his feet, flexing his massive arms, and looking as if he'd never been injured.*

*'Time to get back out there, sir!' one of the kefir soldiers says.*

*'Thanks, soldiers!' Treg says. He sets off after Laughing Cell, at a dead run. You follow, as fast as you can. The white-coated soldiers come too, moving quickly.*

*Treg and the kefir soldiers surround Laughing Cell, who has now swollen up to three times his normal size; his face is glowing an eerie green, and he's still spraying the deadly IgE at everything in his reach.*

*Treg leaps for him and grabs him around the neck, just missing a deadly swipe of the IgE. The kefir soldiers grab one limb each, and they wrestle the IgE out of Laughing Cell's grasp. He howls like a wounded demon.*

*'Good night, soldier,' says Treg. 'Sorry about this. But I did warn you.' He pulls the plug on Laughing Cell and the monstrous B cell deflates, like a balloon.*

*'IgE – they all think they can handle it,' says one of the kefir soldiers.*

*Everyone stands still for a moment, eyes downcast.*

*'Well, we'd better get on with the mop-up,' says the lead kefir soldier. He and Treg salute one another.*

*'You came just in time,' says Treg.*

*'Glad to help, sir,' the kefir soldier replies. 'Just doing our job.'*

*And with that, the three white-coated soldiers turn and jog back to the skin barrier, where the last of the holes are just being sealed up.*

So, as you can see, kefir helps to repair the skin barrier, supports the action of Treg cells in suppressing rogue B cells spraying IgE, and suppresses the allergic reaction. You'll find out more about this amazing probiotic wonder food very soon.

## ✿ GSS TAKEAWAYS ✿

⊕ B cells inside your immune system choose immuno-globulin 'weapons' when faced with an intruder.

⊕ IgE is the 'kamikaze' weapon of the immune system: it may kill cancer cells, but it also causes severe allergic reactions, including eczema.

⊕ TSLP is a communication molecule that alerts other parts of the immune system to an invasion at the body's barrier sites. It also causes the itching that's associated with eczema.

⊕ Left untreated, dry skin can trigger an eczema attack, as scratching an itch drives allergens through the skin barrier.

⊕ Probiotic kefir can halt the allergic march by suppressing the production of IgE inside the immune system.

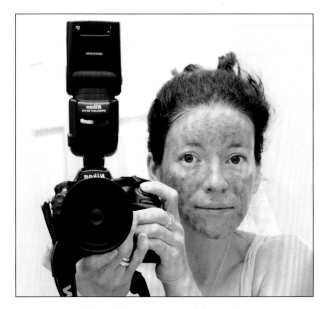

Betsan Evans, rosacea and dermatitis

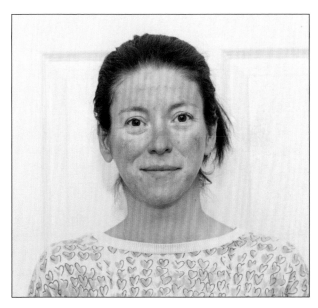

Betsan after 7 months of the GSS. Treatment ongoing.

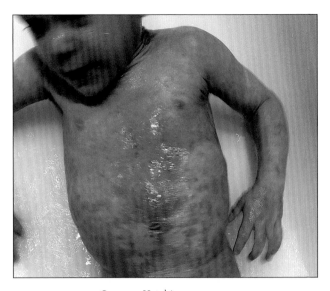

Cameron Hutchinson, eczema

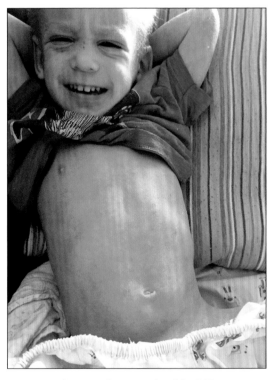

Cameron after 6 months of the GSS

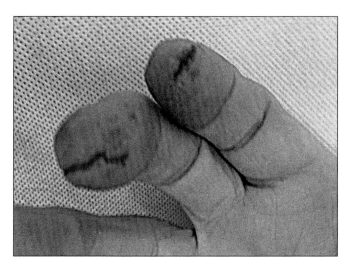

Don Jones, eczema

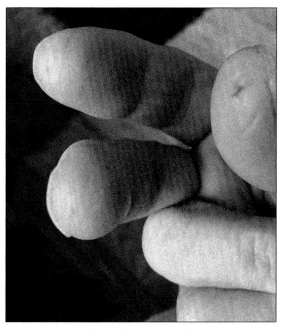

Don's fingers after 2 weeks of the GSS

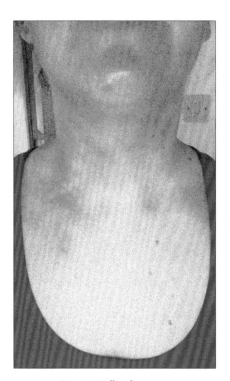

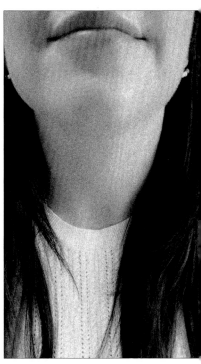

Georgie Hulburd, eczema

Georgie's neck after 9 weeks of the GSS

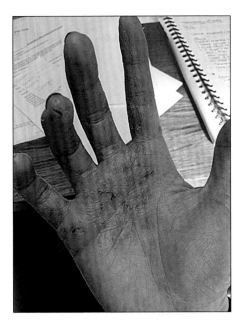

Georgie Hulburd, eczema

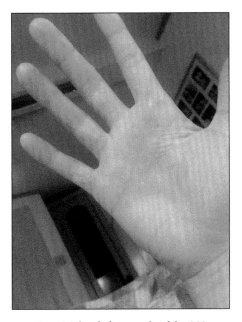

Georgie's hand after 9 weeks of the GSS

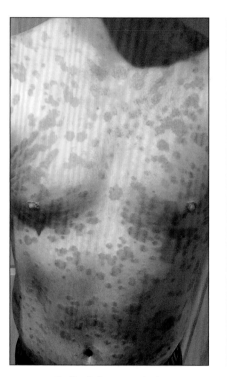

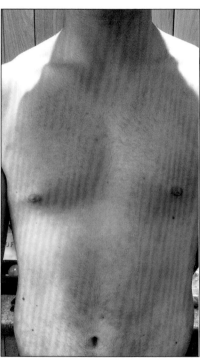

Steffan Roberts, psoriasis       Steffan's chest after 6 months of the GSS

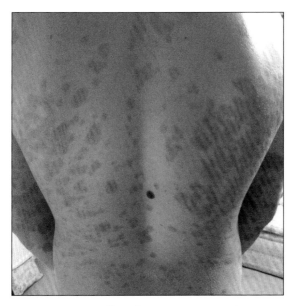

Steffan Roberts, psoriasis

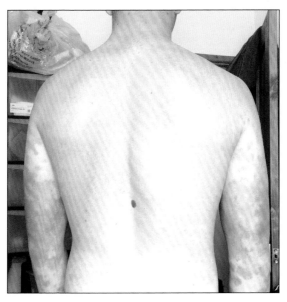

Steffan's back after 6 months of the GSS

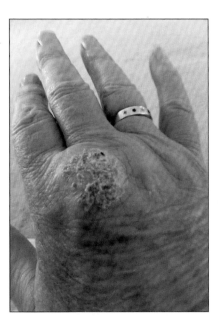

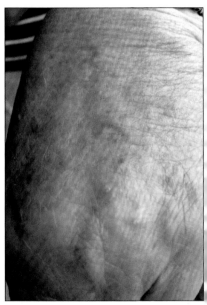

Sherylyn Knight, psoriasis          Sherylyn's hand after 6 months of the GSS

## Chapter 10

# Psoriasis, Rosacea, and Acne

You now have a good idea of what happens inside your immune system when eczema and the allergic march take hold. But what about the other inflammatory skin conditions that we frequently see at Chuckling Goat: psoriasis, rosacea, and acne?

Although these don't follow the allergic march in the same way that eczema does, they *do* all, eventually, respond to the GSS. As you now know, like eczema, psoriasis, and rosacea are autoimmune disorders and acne is an autoimmune spectrum disorder.

**Remember: your skin is just a map of your gut, so whatever you see on the surface of the skin – whether it's eczema, psoriasis, rosacea, or acne – is just a reflection of what's going on in your microbiome.**

You must heal the gut, to heal the skin. The process for this is the same, regardless of the name given to your skin condition. Let's look briefly at each in turn.

# Psoriasis

Psoriasis is an autoimmune condition that affects the skin. Estimated to affect at least 125 million people worldwide, it occurs at various levels of severity, from single inflamed and scaly spots, called 'plaques,' at the elbows or knees to a very severe disease pattern affecting the entire skin.

Most people with psoriasis experience periods of flare-up and remission. Flare-ups are often brought on by external triggers. The 600 participants in a survey by Health Nation in the US reported that they never know when or how often their flare-ups will occur, or their severity.

Sixty-four percent reported that flare-ups occurred at least once a month, and half of those experienced them daily. Thirty-seven percent said their flare-ups lasted for more than three months. The triggers for psoriasis are often difficult to avoid, and the most commonly reported were: stress/anxiety, weather, and infection.[1]

## The psoriatic march

Also, like eczema, psoriasis seldom rides alone. Whereas eczema belongs to the allergic march, psoriasis has its own march: it's often associated with diabetes, depression, inflammatory bowel disease (IBD), and psoriatic arthritis.[2]

Scientists have found that psoriasis is triggered when the immune system produces too many cell-signaling molecules called 'cytokines,' which stimulate other skin cells to create inflammation.[3]

Kefir has been found to suppress this inflammatory response by suppressing cytokine production.[4] This is probably why the GSS produces such strong results with psoriasis. Drinking the kefir reduces inflammation throughout the entire system, while applying the kefir also helps the skin biome re-balance itself and heal naturally.

The diabetes, depression, IBD, and arthritis that accompany psoriasis are all inflammatory conditions. In fact, inflammation is the key culprit here.[5] It stems from microbiome damage, and it manifests differently, in different parts of the body.

Psoriatic inflammation will show itself in the tummy as IBD, in the nervous system as fatigue, in the endocrine system as diabetes, in the behavioral center of the brain as depression, and on the skin as psoriasis.

As you learned earlier, these are not separate issues: they are all symptoms of one autoimmune problem. Just as the symptoms of the allergic march are connected, these psoriatic symptoms are, too. They are leaves of the same microbiome-damage tree. And just as with eczema, the trunk of the tree sits in your gut.

**The GSS can de-rail the psoriatic march, just as it halts the allergic march of eczema. By introducing helpful bacteria into the gut and onto the skin, in the form of kefir, the amount of inflammation in the body is reduced.**

Remember: the most powerful anti-inflammatory is a healthy gut. Reduce the level of inflammation, and the pain in the joints will reduce, as the psoriatic plaques on the skin resolve. All the elements of the psoriatic march are treated at once, and gradually, the symptoms subside.

# Rosacea

Rosacea is a skin disorder characterized by redness and inflammation of the facial skin, mainly on the cheeks, nose, and chin. Often, small blood vessels become visible too. Left untreated, crops of small, inflamed red bumps and pimples can develop.

It's a chronic condition that gradually worsens, and is generally cyclic – flaring up for a period of weeks to months, and then subsiding for a time.

Rosacea is sometimes called 'adult acne,' although it is not the same condition as acne. In the UK, rosacea affects about one in 10 people, and in the US almost 14 million. Sufferers are usually fair-skinned females aged 30–50.

Like eczema and psoriasis, rosacea has been linked with other autoimmune disorders: in this case, type 1 diabetes, celiac disease, multiple sclerosis, and rheumatoid arthritis. There may also be a connection between rosacea and heart disease, depression, migraines, high blood pressure, and high cholesterol,[6] although more research is needed.

The simplest way to understand the possible association is to think of all these issues as a larger autoimmune 'march'; what we call 'rosacea' is simply the way these deeper issues show up on the skin.

## The role of skin mites

Medical research has often pointed to a microscopic skin mite called Demodex folliculorum as a potential factor in rosacea.

We all have Dermodex mites living in the hair follicles of our facial skin – they are part of the skin biome. But it's known that rosacea sufferers have an increased density of them.

However, according to recent research by the National University of Ireland, it's not the mites themselves that trigger rosacea; instead, it's the bacteria that live inside their digestive tracts. The bacterium Bacillus oleronius, which was isolated from inside a Demodex mite, was found to produce molecules that provoke an immune reaction in rosacea patients.

Bacillus oleronius usually live inside Demodex mites in a mutually beneficial relationship. But when the mites die, the bacteria are released and leak into surrounding skin tissues, triggering tissue degradation and inflammation.[7]

Those with rosacea have also been shown to have too much of an anti-microbial peptide called cathelicidin. This is a small protein in the body's defense system, normally known for its role in protecting the skin against infection. But in rosacea patients, the overload of peptides causes an increase in inflammation.[8]

Although in its early stages rosacea may look less severe than psoriasis, on the farm we've found that it's a stubborn condition that's difficult to resolve. Tackling rosacea with the GSS requires time, patience, and dedication to the recommended dietary changes.

## GSS SUCCESS STORY

*A dermatologist told me I had rosacea and dermatitis. I'd been suffering since 2010/11, but recently it became totally extreme, covering all of my face. It was not only physically painful – with itchiness, burning, and dryness – but emotionally painful, too. It hit my self-esteem and really got me down. I thought I looked like a monster.*

*I tried a massive detox and extreme clean diets, but my skin just got worse and worse. I started losing faith in all kinds of medicine and healthy diets. Then I discovered Chuckling Goat. I placed my first order of kefir in May, 2016, and I'm now on my seventh month.*

*To begin with, nothing much happened – my skin was still the same, although I'd been keeping to a dairy-, gluten-, and sugar-free diet. In August 2016, I started noticing changes: the redness was reducing, there were no more boil-like breakouts popping up on my face. My skin seemed to be calming down! People started saying things like: 'Betsan, your face is getting better,' and 'the shape of your face is going back to how it's supposed to be.'*

*It's truly overwhelming, the transformation that's happened in the last two months. I still have little blemishes on my face, but I'm now able to cover them with make up and feel normal again. Last week I had a realization: I'm not in pain anymore and that feels strange. I feel very emotional.*

*Although I'm not totally cured, I know that by drinking kefir every day and following a clean eating diet, along with regular exercise and fresh air, I will win the war against my skin condition.*

*Thank you Shann, for your continuous coaching. You are the only one out of all the alternative health experts who has stuck by me and not given up on helping me.*

*Diolch o galon (thank you)*

BETSAN EVANS

(See photographs in the colour section.)

## Acne

We usually associate acne with the teenage years, but dermatologists are finding that adult-onset acne is becoming increasingly common in people, especially women, in their 20s, 30s, 40s, and even 50s.

**Adult-onset acne is on the rise in the UK. A 2015 study of 92 private dermatology clinics found an eyebrow-raising 200 percent increase in the number of people seeking specialist acne treatment.**

'It is like an epidemic,' says Dr. Stefanie Williams, medical director of Eudelo (European Dermatology London). 'We have so many sufferers (in this country). It is important to acknowledge that this is a skin disease. It is not normal and not a rite of passage.'[9]

Acne is caused by the over-production of sebum (oil) in the sebaceous glands – tiny glands near skin's surface – usually driven by changes in hormone levels. The condition develops when the skin's hair follicles get blocked with sebum and dead skin cells, leading to blackheads.

If the follicle stays blocked, it can become inflamed, resulting in spots and cysts. Sometimes, a bacterium called Propionibacterium acnes (P. acnes for short) that usually lives harmlessly on the skin, grows inside the follicles, which also contributes to the inflammation.

## The latest science

Like the other autoimmune skin conditions we've been looking at, acne has been linked to the microbiome by very recent research. A study dated August 2015 states that 'An imbalance in the microbial community may cause pathological conditions... of the skin such as... acne.'[10]

Women are five times more likely than men to be affected by late-onset acne. Specialists variously blame this on fluctuating hormones during pregnancy, the menstrual cycle, changing methods of contraception, and increased amounts of stress in women's daily lives.[11]

Dr. Williams also blames the surge in adult acne on choosing the wrong kind of skincare. 'Those in their thirties or forties who start to see lines and wrinkles begin investing in anti-aging skincare regimes,' she notes. 'These creams can be very rich, and overload the skin and cause acne, in acne-prone individuals.'[12]

## The role of stress

Low-level changes in stress have long been linked to problem skin, because the body's stress hormone (cortisol) contributes to breakouts. Dr. Nick Lowe, consultant dermatologist at the Cranley Clinic in London, believes it's this stress that's fueling the rise in adult acne, especially in women who are working full-time while raising families.

He says, 'There are so many triggers: perceived shortness of time… women being pressured at both work and home.'[13]

But how does stress actually cause acne? (Or flare-ups of eczema, psoriasis, or rosacea?) After treating hundreds of patients over the years with these conditions, US dermatologist Dr. Flor A. Mayoral has seen how it can aggravate the skin.

When a person becomes stressed, the level of cortisol rises. This in turn causes an increase in oil production, which can lead to oily skin, acne, and other related skin problems. Dr. Mayoral noted that even patients with skin that's not affected by acne tends to develop temporary stress-related breakouts due to increased oil production.[14]

## GSS SUCCESS STORY

*I purchased your kefir 21-day course last month, and I just wanted to let you know about my positive results!! I've been suffering with blemishes for the past year, which escalated into full-blown acne this summer.*

*I was at a complete loss as to what to do until I stumbled upon an article that talked about how one's gut could affect one's skin and suggested your goat's milk. Since completing your GSS course, my skin has improved in leaps and bounds and my digestion is definitely a lot better*

*Thank you so much!! :)*

VICTORIA LENTON

## Drawbacks of current treatment

To date, scientists have made limited progress in developing new strategies for treating acne. Dermatologists' arsenal of anti-acne tools – benzoyl peroxide, antibiotics, and isotretinoin – hasn't expanded in decades.

Most severe cases of acne don't respond to antibiotics[15] and isotretinoin (widely marketed as Accutane when first released), which is commonly used to treat severe acne, can have severe side effects, including headaches, joint pain, and liver damage. It is strongly contra-indicated for pregnancy as it can harm a fetus, causing craniofacial, cardiac, and central nervous system defects.[16]

## Probiotics can help

Although everyone's skin biome contains P. acnes, the bacterium that's believed to play a role in acne, around one in five people are fortunate enough to develop only an occasional pimple. So what's their secret? Hopefully, with your new knowledge of yourself as a holobiont, you're now shouting out: *acne, like psoriasis, eczema, and rosacea, is the result of an imbalance in the microbiome.*

And sure enough, scientists have found that not *all* strains of P. acnes bacteria trigger pimples. One strain may actually keep it healthy and clear. According to scientist Huiying Li at the David Geffen School of Medicine at UCLAL, 'This P. acnes strain may protect the skin, much like yogurt's live bacteria helps defend the gut from harmful bugs. Our next step will be to investigate whether a probiotic cream can block bad bacteria from invading the skin, and prevent pimples before they start.'[17]

I couldn't have put it better myself! **The GSS implements this cutting-edge approach to acne by using a probiotic cream.**

Along with drinking kefir to reduce levels of inflammation in the body, the GSS includes the use of kefir-based skincare, which allows the beneficial strains of bacteria living in the skin biome to out-pace the 'bad' strains that cause pimples.

According to research conducted at Leeds Metropolitan University in the UK, thyme essential oil is more effective against acne bacteria than benzoyl peroxide,[18] without any of the drying and redness that chemical can cause. Which is why we combine thyme essential oil with tea tree essential oil in our Break-Out range (*see Resources section*).

Consuming probiotics has also been found to lower levels of stress-induced hormones in the system, calming the conditions that cause acne flares. This may have the additional benefit of helping to reduce anxiety and depression.[19]

Emerging research suggests there may also be a link between a low-glycemic diet and an improvement in acne.[20] This is why we've made the consumption of low GI foods one of the habits of the GSS (you'll find out more about these in Part IV).

# ✺ GSS TAKEAWAYS ✺

✢ Psoriasis is often accompanied by a 'psoriatic march' of other conditions, including diabetes, depression, IBD, and arthritis. These are inflammatory conditions that respond well to the GSS.

✢ Rosacea can be accompanied by type 1 diabetes, celiac disease, multiple sclerosis, and rheumatoid arthritis. It is the most difficult skin condition to shift with the GSS, but will respond over time.

✢ Adult acne is on the rise, and antibiotics are relatively ineffective as a solution. Probiotics as used in the GSS help to restore the skin biome and prevent harmful acne bacteria from taking over.

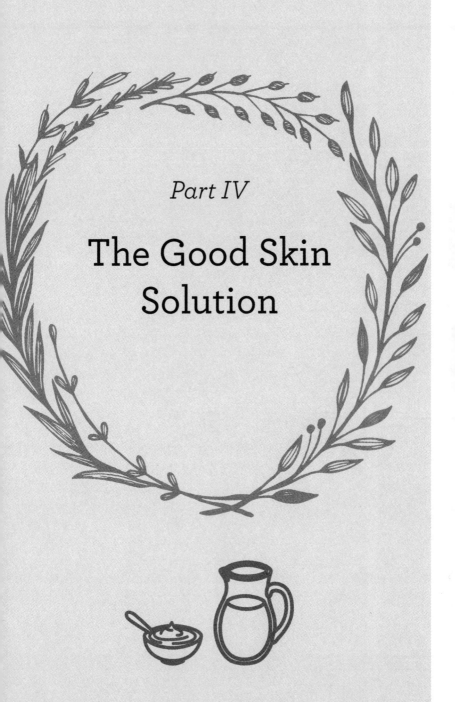

*Part IV*

# The Good Skin Solution

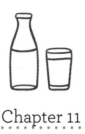

## Chapter 11

# Kefir: a Probiotic Powerhouse

Earlier in the book I explained how a probiotic product called kefir, made using milk from the goats on our family farm, helped save my husband's life when he contracted an MRSA 'superbug.'

I also described how the kefir-based skincare range I subsequently developed has helped thousands of people with eczema, psoriasis, acne, and rosacea. Kefir is the linchpin of the GSS, so let's find out more about it.

## Kefir and the immune system

In Chapter 9, you learned how kefir can work with our immune cells to fend off an eczema attack. In fact, scientific studies have found that kefir can halt eczema, and the other conditions of the allergic march, by acting on the immune system in the following three ways:

1.  By suppressing the production of IgE antibodies.[1]

2.  By preventing allergy-producing antigens from passing through the intestinal wall.[2]

3.  By enhancing the action of protective Treg cells.[3]

Having spent some time on the front lines of your immune system border patrol, you now understand a bit more about why these actions are so crucial. So let's now find out exactly what kefir *is* and where it originated.

## What's so special about kefir?

Kefir is a potent drink made by fermenting milk with a living kefir culture that contains multiple strains of beneficial bacteria and yeast. It has long been known that ingesting such live microorganisms – which are known as 'probiotics' – can aid digestion and boost immune system function. In recent years, as scientists have learned more about the role of probiotics in the human microbiome, interest in them has soared.

But all probiotics are not created equal. Liquid probiotics, which contain bacteria living and thriving in their own medium, increasing in strength and numbers over time, are more powerful than products containing dried or dehydrated probiotic, in which the bacteria die off over time.

**If you suffer from eczema, psoriasis, rosacea, or acne, you need the exponentially greater strength of a multi-strain probiotic like kefir, whose vast number of beneficial bacteria and yeasts work as a symbiotic whole.**

It's far more effective than popping a probiotic pill or powder that will generally contain *just one or two strains* of good bacteria.

And, crucially, the bacteria in kefir is 'non-transient,' which means that many of the bacterial strains survive the digestive process and actually reach the large intestine, where they can achieve long-term benefits. This is different than 'live' yogurt, which contains 'transient' bacteria that's killed off by stomach acid during digestion.

## What's the best type of kefir?

Kefir can be made from cow, goat, oat, or almond milk. You can also make water kefir with water kefir grains, but this is much less powerful than milk kefir, and you need to consume more as a daily dose.

If you suffer from a skin condition caused by an autoimmune disorder, like those covered in this book, you should choose kefir that's dairy milk-based, because it has been shown that dairy products boost the effectiveness of probiotics.[4]

Choose kefir made with goat's milk rather than cow's milk, too, because studies show that goat's milk is more beneficial to human health than cow's milk, and much less allergenic.[5] Cow's milk is a known trigger for eczema, and should be avoided by anyone working with a skin condition; we'll discuss this in greater detail later.

**Live, active goat's milk kefir returns those good bugs to where they need to be inside your body – and repairs the damage to**

your microbiome that's been caused over time by antibiotics, sugar, stress, and antimicrobial products.[6]

## GSS SUCCESS STORY

*The 'before and after' photos I've sent you don't really show the mess I was in: the patches of infected eczema on my hand and knee were thick and crusty, swollen, and constantly oozing muck. One of your girls kindly suggested soaking dressings in kefir before covering the areas with a bandage when I was going out, as my clothing would stick to them. That was a marvellous tip.*

*I'm now on my fourth/fifth course of drinking kefir and using the creams and soap. I can't express what a difference all this has made to me, and my friends and family are astonished. I'd been given four courses of antibiotics to try to stem the infection, and was using steroids every day.*

*Once I received my order from Chuckling Goat, I washed the infected areas twice a day with the Break-Out Kefir Lotion and bathed every three days with the bath melts. Previously, I'd tried so many things and spent so much money, only for the eczema to return. But this time, I'm so confident that won't happen: the skin has renewed itself.*

*I actually wore a light pair of trousers all day today, without tearing myself to bits – for the first time in four months! My legs aren't 100 percent clear yet, but we're almost there. Thank you all for your help and support over the last six months.*

*The transformation continues and I've recommended you to so many people, I've lost count – among them shop assistants*

*who've seen my hand transform from a weeping mess to nearly
perfect, and members of my family and friends.*

*A big thank you to all you 'girls,' especially for your patience
when I've asked so many questions. You've all made this possible.*

SHERYLYN KNIGHT

(See photographs in the colour section.)

## How is kefir made?

Kefir is made by placing kefir 'grains' into a vessel, adding
fresh milk, and then allowing the mixture to stand at room
temperature for 24–36 hours until a thick, creamy drink is
produced. Kefir 'grains' are not grains like wheat, but living
clusters of yeasts and bacteria that resemble small, soft pieces
of white coral.

The grains consist of casein and gelatinous colonies of
microorganisms that are grown together symbiotically, and
then used to produce a uniquely powerful, tart, and fizzy
substance.

The kefir grains ferment the milk, incorporating their own
'friendly' bacteria to create a 'live' cultured product. At
the end of the process, the kefir grains are removed with a
strainer, the resulting drinking kefir is poured into another
vessel, and the grains are added to a new batch of milk,
beginning the fermentation process all over again.

Kefir grains cannot be manufactured – they can only grow
from other kefir grains. Properly looked after, kefir grains will

live indefinitely, reproducing and continually doubling in size as they grow.

## Where did kefir come from?

No one knows where the very *first* kefir grain came from. It's a mystery, lost in the probiotic food's 1,900 year-old history, which began in the Caucasus Mountains of Eastern Europe (occupied today by Russia, Georgia, Azerbaijan, and Armenia).

For centuries, little was known about kefir outside this region, despite the fact that the famous Venetian explorer Marco Polo mentioned kefir in his writings after traveling there in the 1260s.

The shepherd inhabitants of the Caucasus guarded their kefir grains jealously, calling them 'The Grains of the Prophet,' and refusing to give them away to outsiders. Grains were passed down as dowries within families, and although outsiders were occasionally given some of the fizzy beverage to drink, no one was allowed to handle the kefir grains or learn the secrets of kefir's production. As a result, kefir remained unknown in the rest of the world for many centuries.

## How did kefir use spread?

In the late 19th century, news reached Russia that kefir was being used successfully to treat tuberculosis and intestinal and stomach diseases. Doctors there began to look seriously at its purported health benefits.

In 1908, the Nobel prize-winning Russian-born zoologist and microbiologist Elie Metchnikoff, best known for his pioneering research in immunology, became curious about the longevity of mountain peasants in Bulgaria. Their lifespan was an unusually high 87 years, and Metchnikoff theorized that their consumption of milk fermented by bacilli (a bacteria) was a key factor in this.

Despite these tantalizing scientific developments, kefir was still very difficult to find, as it was impossible to produce without the kefir grains themselves. Determined to establish a source of the elusive grains in order to make a scientific study, members of the 'All Russian Physicians' Society' approached two brothers named Blandov, owners of the large Moscow Dairy in the town of Kislovodsk, in the northern Caucasus.

## Irina and the prince

What happened next is straight out of the pages of a romance novel. Nikolai Blandov recruited a beautiful young female employee named Irina Sakharova, and sent her off, along with an armed guard, to the court of a Caucasian prince named Bek-Mirza Barchorov. Irina's instructions were to charm the prince into giving her some kefir grains for the study.

The prince was indeed enchanted by the lovely Irina, but he was too afraid of violating religious law – which protected the Grains of the Prophet from outsiders – to give her any grains. Admitting defeat, Irina and her escort party began the return trip to Kislovodsk.

But Bek-Mirza Barchorov was unable to forget Irina. Conveniently, there was a local custom that allowed a bridegroom to kidnap his chosen bride, and so the prince sent the men of a local mountain tribe to capture Irina. After dragging her back to his court, he proposed marriage. Irina bravely remained silent, which bought her enough time for the Blandov brothers to organize an armed rescue party to come to her aid.

They succeeded in their rescue mission. After Irina was returned home, Bek-Mirza Barchorov was brought before the Russian tsar, Nicholas II, to answer for his actions. The tsar ruled that in compensation for the kidnapping, and other insults to her person that she was forced to endure, the prince must give Irina 10 pounds of kefir grains.

## Growing popularity

In 1973, when Irina Sakharova was 85 years old, the Minister of Food and Industry of the Soviet Union sent her a letter, thanking her for bringing kefir to the Russian people. Hospitals in the former USSR used kefir to treat conditions ranging from atherosclerosis, allergic disease, metabolic and digestive disorders, cancer, and gastric disorders.

Today, kefir is produced on a large scale in former Soviet countries. Late in the 20th century, kefir accounted for between 64 and 80 percent of total fermented milk sales in Russia, with production of over 1.2 million tons per year in 1988.

The production of kefir has since spread from the former USSR, and the drink is now regularly consumed in North America, South America, Europe, and Australia. And now, finally, kefir has reached the UK.

## ✿ GSS TAKEAWAYS ✿

⊕ Kefir is a powerful probiotic drink that originated in Eastern Europe's Caucasus Mountains.

⊕ Goat's milk is the best base for kefir, as it increases the power of the probiotics.

⊕ The most powerful kefir is made with real kefir grains.

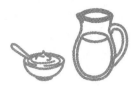

## Chapter 12

# Kefir and the GSS

Now that you know more about kefir, and how it works inside the immune system, let's talk about how it can help your skin condition as part of the GSS. Here on the farm, we've found that the most effective way to use kefir is to drink it – which heals the gut biome – *and* apply it to the skin in the form of cleansers and lotions – which heals the skin biome.

This combination of probiotic oral and topical immunotherapy, together with dietary changes, makes up the Good Skin Solution (GSS); you'll find out how to follow the GSS in the next chapter. But first, here's a quick recap of what you've learned so far:

1. Eczema, psoriasis, rosacea, and acne are autoimmune disorders, not simple skin conditions.

2. Your immune system mainly sits in the gut, and is controlled by your microbiome.

3. Your microbiome can be damaged by antibiotics, sugar, stress, and environmental toxins.

4. An autoimmune disorder that's showing up on your skin can be resolved by simultaneously applying kefir topically, to rebalance your skin biome, and taking it internally to aid your gut biome.

That's an outline of the problem, and the solution. Your gut and skin biomes can be helped by probiotic immunotherapy. And kefir, as the probiotic with the widest range of good bacteria, provides the boost they need

## 'Levels' of microbiome damage

When increasing numbers of people began to drink our goat's milk kefir and use our kefir-based skincare, I realized something – previously, those clients had had no one to ask for advice. Nobody else was doing what we were doing; we were innovating a new process. We had to quickly learn our way around this new health terrain.

We started to log the cumulative, real-world experiences of our clients as they followed our GSS. They reported their results back to us after taking one or more 21-day 'courses' of our kefir, simultaneously applying our lotions and cleansers to their skin, and adopting our recommended dietary changes (coming up in the next chapter).

Some clients were seeing immediate results; for others, improvement took a little longer. Out of this experience we developed our own definitions of the various manifestations of microbiome damage on the skin. For simplicity's sake, we now describe these as 'levels.'

The information below will help you determine the 'level' of your microbiome damage, in terms of your eczema, psoriasis, acne, or rosacea. It also explains what you can expect when you adopt the GSS.

## *Level one – mild*

✦ Eczema, psoriasis, and acne of fairly recent origin

Clients whose skin disturbances (most often eczema, but sometimes just described as a 'skin rash' or 'spots') had started within the previous two years or less, often found that they cleared up permanently after three 21-day courses of kefir, and the simultaneous application of kefir skincare.

Many also adopted the GSS dietary changes, but found that they could safely backslide on these once their skin issue had resolved. (As you'll soon discover, though, it's beneficial to eat along GSS lines permanently, for general microbiome health, lowered inflammation, and weight loss!)

Often, these skin problems appeared to date from a course of antibiotics. It seemed to us that these issues indicated a fairly mild level of microbiome damage, recently incurred.

Level-one clients often experienced a 'detox' reaction around days 3–5 of their first kefir course, as the probiotic began to do its spring-cleaning work inside the gut. Symptoms could include nausea, headaches, wind, bloating, or a temporary worsening of the skin condition. These detox symptoms generally cleared around days 8–9, after which clients reported feeling a surge in energy and wellbeing, a suppression of sugar cravings, and a feeling of calm.

Although the majority of our clients began drinking our kefir to deal with their skin issues, most of them found it also had the pleasant side effect of helping resolve gut issues such as IBS, diverticulitis, bloating, cramping, and other gastric problems. These tended to resolve fairly early on in the process, even before clients saw results on their skin.

## Level two – moderate

✤ Eczema, psoriasis, and acne of 2–10 years' duration

At this level of microbiome damage, clients definitely needed three consecutive 21-day courses of kefir before seeing much improvement in their skin condition. They also had to continue the kefir skincare beyond the kefir course, and follow the GSS dietary habits stringently.

As well as an initial 'detox' reaction around days 3–5 of the first kefir course, we noticed that a lot of level-two folk experienced a second detox, toward the end of their second course of kefir. A frequently reported symptom was a flare-up of the skin condition for a brief period of time, accompanied by fatigue. The detox symptoms generally subsided by the beginning of the third course of kefir.

The start of the third course was also the time when, commonly, clients' skin symptoms began to fade. They also reported a reduction in allergies and hay fever. Many said they felt energetic, healthy, and upbeat; and of course, they were thrilled when their skin finally began to clear!

We found that once their skin condition had cleared, level-two clients could stop taking kefir daily, and move to taking a quarterly booster course in the spring, summer, autumn, and winter. This tops up the good bugs inside the gut, enabling them to cope with the damage that antibiotics, stress, sugar, and use of antimicrobial products have done in the meantime.

We also found it was important that level-two clients followed the GSS dietary habits for at least a year, or their condition would tend to re-appear.

## Level three – severe

✤ Eczema from birth; rosacea; psoriasis and acne of 10+ years' duration

These clients generally needed to drink our kefir and use the skincare continually for at least six months in order to see strong initial results. They also needed to follow the GSS dietary habits stringently. To prevent backsliding, all three elements of the GSS had to be followed indefinitely.

Similar to level two, clients with severe microbiome damage nearly always experienced an initial, early detox and at least one more detox period toward the end of the second course of drinking kefir. The rule seemed to be the more severe the microbiome damage, the more difficult the detox.

Although we saw a few cases of rosacea resolve rapidly within nine weeks, this condition has proven much more stubborn and difficult to shift. Clients with rosacea tend to report that it has lingered inside their system for a decade or more, so the level of microbiome disturbance is deep-seated. Eczema, psoriasis, and acne that have persisted for more than 10 years also required similar treatment.

At this level of microbiome damage, clients also reported sleeplessness, constant, unbearable itching, and even emotional disorders, from the assault on the behavioral center of the brain as the immune system turns on itself.

The resulting autoimmune issues will almost always include depression, anxiety, and fatigue, as well as gastric disorders such as constipation or IBS. Level-three clients' skin lesions were sometimes so disfiguring that they avoided going outside, and didn't want to be seen.

We've seen some extraordinary results with level-three clients, which they have described as 'life-changing.' Clients who've had dysbiosis (an imbalance in gut bacteria) since birth – like my little friend Cameron – have never had a properly functioning microbiome. Being able to help people in so much distress is one of the most satisfying things I've ever done.

The kefir has a lot of work to do at level-three damage! This is why the system appears to need ongoing doses of good kefir probiotics, from the inside and outside, as well as constant monitoring of the diet, to keep it in good order.

## GSS SUCCESS STORY

*About a year ago, I was suffering from eczema on my hands and wrists that was not only very itchy but causing lots of open cracks and sores due to where it was on my body. I was also having trouble with my gut and spent a lot of mornings gurgling and churning my way through until lunchtime, even on a good breakfast!*

*Having heard Shann Jones's fascinating talk on the radio, I went onto the website and bought a course of kefir, as well as some bath melts and facial soap. Can I just say a big thank you! Not only did it sort my gut out, I also felt so much more energized in the mornings.*

*My eczema also totally cleared up over the next couple of months and hasn't come back since! I'm a big believer that the kefir had a profound and positive effect on my overall health, and I've been recommending it to fellow eczema sufferers as an alternative to the harsh over-the-counter treatments ever since.*

VICTORIA POTTERTON

## Working with nature

Our clients were becoming 'experts of their own wellness.' Once they reached a plateau of wellbeing, their skin was looking good, and they were feeling calm, happy, and full of energy, they would readily notice if their state began to slip downhill again. They would know instantly that it was time for a top-up course of kefir.

Once we've re-seeded our microbiome with the good bacteria in kefir, we need to be mindful that those seeds are delicate, and need time to grow. A microbiome that's been out of balance for decades is going to take some serious work; that ecosystem platform will have to endure major serious wobbles before it stabilizes into a new, healthier pattern.

Nature takes time to weave her magic, but if you work with her, you *will* see results.

Microbiome damage doesn't occur overnight, and it won't be resolved overnight. But over time, the microbiome can be rehabilitated through the GSS, and you'll see that outcome on your skin.

### ✺ GSS TAKEAWAYS ✺

⊕ Microbiome damage that shows up on the skin can be organized into three levels: level one (mild); level two (moderate), level three (severe).

⊕ Your level of microbiome damage will determine how long you need to follow the GSS before you see initial results, as well as how long you will need to continue the program to maintain those results.

## Chapter 13

# The GSS in Seven Daily Habits

So, it's now time to put some microbiome-friendly practices in place – and start the process of healing your skin condition – by following the GSS.

As someone who has moved continents and adjusted to an entirely new way of life, I know that sometimes change can feel overwhelming. So I've broken down the GSS into seven simple daily habits that can easily be incorporated into your life.

Here's an outline of each GSS habit; in the following chapters, you'll discover the science behind them, and find out why and how they can help your skin.

**Habit #1: Drink goat's milk kefir**

**Habit #2: Use goat's milk kefir skincare**

**Habit #3: Drink bone broth**

Habit #4: Replace sugar with stevia

Habit #5: Eat goat dairy

Habit #6: Choose slow-burning foods

Habit #7: Go for good fats

## How the GSS works

The GSS is centered on a 21-day 'course' of drinking goat's milk kefir and using goat's milk kefir-based skincare (habits #1 and 2).

**The good probiotic bugs in the drinking kefir and the kefir-based skincare do most of the heavy lifting to promote the healing of the gut and skin biomes. But it's important to support those changes with what you eat.**

If you regularly consume refined sugar, for example, you're killing off those good bugs as fast as you put them into your system. So habits #3–7 are designed to replace biome-harming foods with biome-friendly alternatives.

Start drinking the kefir and using the kefir skincare on day one of the course. Then, every few days, introduce one of the other five habits. By the end of your first kefir course, you'll have seamlessly incorporated the entire GSS into your daily life.

The duration of your kefir 'treatment' – i.e. the number of 21-day courses you'll need before you see an improvement in your skin condition – will depend on your level of microbiome damage (*see Chapter 12*).

I suggest you continue using kefir-based skincare twice daily, even after your skin has improved. Your skin biome is continually assaulted by harsh weather, drying central heating, allergens, pollution, and toxins in the chemicals that you encounter every day, so it needs the probiotic boost, moisturizing, and natural healing that kefir skincare provides on an ongoing basis. And for the sake of your skin and general health, habits #3–7 should become a permanent part of your diet.

## Tips for following the GSS

As you read about the GSS in the following chapters, you'll see that the whole process is designed to *add* things into your existing lifestyle, so you'll more easily be able to let go of the things that are damaging your microbiome.

### Adopt one habit at a time

I don't call the GSS a 'diet,' as I believe that has a harsh, restrictive ring. Most of us are already working hard, so we don't want to be told to give up the nice yummy things we eat to make the day bearable – it's just too much!

However, you may find that once you add something in, you'll more readily let go of the 'baddies' that are harming your microbiome. For example, adding the natural sweetener stevia into your diet (habit #4) makes it easier to let go of sugar. Or start enjoying goat's milk, cheese, and butter (habit #5) so you can drop the allergenic cow dairy that may be making your skin condition worse.

Be gentle with yourself as you start to follow the GSS. Like a good parent, be firm but fair instead of harsh and critical. I like to think of my subconscious as a grumpy toddler that needs to be lured into doing things by the promise of little treats and rewards.

Think 'baby steps,' and adopt one habit at a time.

## Download your GSS health journal

In order to help you do this, we've created a free downloadable 21-day GSS health journal. It's full of GSS habit prompts, inspirational quotes to keep you going, and a chart on which you can keep a detailed record of the health changes you're experiencing each day.

If you're going to become an expert of your own wellness, it's important that you become your own case study! You can download the journal at:

https://chucklinggoat.co.uk/gss/gss-health-journal.pdf

**For more recipes, hints, and helpful tips about ways to put the Seven Daily Habits of the GSS to work in your own life, please see my blog site, thefarmerswife.wales.**

## Take care of yourself

If you're a parent or a carer, I'd like to offer you a challenge: what if you were to take care of yourself with the same degree of wonderful attention and nurturing that you lavish on your loved ones? Often, we treat ourselves with a very different standard of loving-kindness than we reserve for those we cherish. Turn this same standard of nurturing on yourself, and see what a difference it makes. Be kind to yourself for a change!

Self-care is actually one of the best things you can do for your family and those you love. Nurturers are like wells, and needy people are constantly coming to dip out of that well. Each new crisis that needs to be addressed lowers the water level in your personal well.

But if you don't do anything to refill it, it will soon run dry – and the next person who comes to you for nurturing will find there isn't anything left! If you run out of energy, resources, patience, and good health, you won't be able to care for your loved ones.

## Ways to refill your well

So spend some time thinking how you can refill your own well. Here are some ideas:

- **Take a walk** in a wood, breathe deeply, and look up at the leaves.

- **Take a long bath** containing healing bath melts (*see Resources section*)

- **Get up a bit earlier** in the morning and in a gratitude journal, write down three things that make you happy.

- **Take yourself out** to the cinema, or sign up for a pottery course. Get your hands dirty!

- **Plan some time** in the evening to sit down and soak your feet in a tub of warm water; add a few drops of a healing essential oil like lavender or rosemary to refresh your skin and your nervous system.

Time spent on yourself is not wasted – it's a necessary exercise to refill the well. And the people who rely on you will benefit the most.

## Adopt the 80–20 rule

Here's another top tip while you're instituting the new habits of the GSS: on special occasions, cut yourself some slack. Here on the farm, we're big believers in the 80–20 rule: namely, that if we're 'good' for 80 percent of the time, we can have treats during the other 20 percent. Anything harsher than this, I find, is simply unrealistic. This is a marathon, not a sprint!

Be practical about what you can accomplish – overwhelm is the enemy. We're busy on the farm, and I can't afford to feel hungry, grumpy, or deprived. I need to feel full, happy, and contented after I eat, because I need to bring my best self to my family and my work, every day.

**The GSS involves making long-term, positive changes to your eating patterns that will support the health of your entire system and help reboot your microbiome.**

## GSS SUCCESS STORY

*My husband Don and I came to your open day on the farm in May; Don visited again in June, just two weeks after he'd started taking your kefir. On the second visit, he showed you his hands, which before the kefir had been very bad with what's been diagnosed as eczema. The change was incredible.*

*We are still trying to eradicate the eczema – so far, it's hanging on – but at least Don's no longer in pain, and can use his hands without them bleeding.*

*I bought a course of kefir too and am sold on it – it's like turning the clock back 10 years! I was having days of feeling extremely fatigued, but those are now almost a thing of the past. And generally, I just feel great. It's amazing stuff.*

*Kind regards, and we'll see you at another open day soon.*

YVONNE JONES

(See photographs in the colour section.)

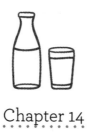

## Chapter 14

# GSS Habit #1: Drink Goat's Milk Kefir

For 21 days, drink 170 ml (6 fl oz) of goat's milk kefir, first thing in the morning, before eating. This gives the good bugs in the kefir the clearest possible run at your gut, without food getting involved. (The kefir probiotics adhere to the lining of the gut, where they will battle it out with the bad bugs.) It's fine to have tea, coffee, or hot water with lemon first.

You can buy goat's milk kefir ready to drink – Chuckling Goat's kefir can be ordered directly from the farm and shipped to your door (*see Resources section*) – or purchase your own kefir grains and follows the preparation instructions that come with them.

This therapeutic 21-day 'course' of probiotics will reboot your microbiome, thus strengthening your immune system over time, so it can resist anything that's thrown at it. It will also shore it up against ongoing attacks.

As you now know, your microbiome is continually assaulted by sugar, antibiotics, stress, and environmental toxins. Even if you haven't taken antibiotics prescribed by a doctor, you'll still have been getting a slow and constant leach of them through the food chain and ground water.

# How long should I take kefir?

It usually takes a minimum of nine weeks (three back-to-back 21-day courses of kefir) before results are seen. Once you've achieved the desired result and your skin is looking good, you can decide whether or not to continue taking kefir in the long term. If you decide to stop, I suggest you have a minimum of one 21-day booster course at the beginning of each season, to keep your immune defenses up.

Remember, it's a matter of keeping the population of good bugs in your gut high and taking up the space, so the bad bugs can't get a toehold.

## An energy boost

You can turn your daily dose of kefir into a nice little ritual – my family and employees make kefir smoothies together every morning, in the farmhouse kitchen (*see recipes below*). Kefir taken early in the day gets your brain off to a great start. The reason for this is that kefir contains lactate, which is your body's preferred energy source.

Lactate causes cells in the brain to release more noradrenaline, a hormone and neurotransmitter that's fundamental for brain function. Lactate is produced naturally in the body – for example, when the muscles are at work, which reinforces the connection between exercise and wellbeing. In the brain, it's regarded as an energy source that can be delivered to neurons as fuel to keep them working when brain activity increases.[1]

Note that lactate, or lactic acid, is different than *lactose*, which is an allergen. Kefir is *lactose-free*, as all the lactose in the milk is consumed during the fermentation process. So if you are lactose intolerant, kefir is safe for you to take. In fact, kefir is recommended to help with the symptoms of lactose-intolerance.[2]

Try to source kefir that is unflavored, because sugar and fruit flavorings will degrade the power of the probiotics. And make sure that it's been made with real kefir grains, rather than a powdered kefir starter culture. For those with an autoimmune skin condition and/or allergies, goat's milk kefir is preferable to cow's milk kefir; find out why in habit #5.

## Guidelines for making your own kefir

If you decide to make kefir at home, it's important to observe the following 'best practice' food safety precautions to make sure it's safe for consumption:

1.  Ferment your kefir until the pH is below 4.5 – this is the level at which most bacterial pathogens are unable to survive. pH meters are readily available online.

2.  Test a batch of your finished drinking kefir regularly at a public health laboratory that offers a standard microbiological food safety screen for live culture products. This will ensure that you're not reusing grains that have become contaminated.

Whenever you reuse a live culture (which is what kefir grains are), you run the risk of 'bacteriophage' contamination. Bacteriophages (or 'phages') are viruses that infect bacteria. They are found in ecosystems where bacteria are commonly found, including man-made ecological niches such as food fermentation vats[3] or jars.

Bacteriophages can turn harmless bacteria into agents of disease, by transferring to them genes that produce toxic substances.[4] These bacteria are then able to infect humans and cause food poisoning and other potentially deadly diseases. At Chuckling Goat we have our kefir regularly tested by a microbiology lab to ensure that it's free from phage or pathogen infection.

I recommend that if you make kefir at home, you do the same! Otherwise you run the risk of a phage infection getting into your grains, which if you continue to use them, will increase over time. As you cannot sterilize the grains themselves, this is a problem. You will have to discard your grains and start over.

**Important note:** the client feedback and results reported in this book reflect the consumption of Chuckling Goat kefir, which we make on the farm. They are not representative of any other kefir, produced commercially or domestically.

Kefir grains are living organisms with unique bio-profiles, and they are not all guaranteed to be the same. Our kefir grains have been DNA-strained and trialed for efficacy by Aberystwyth University in Wales. I cannot personally speak for the efficacy of any other kefir, made with other grains.

## Kefir smoothie recipes

Goat's milk kefir is – let's say this politely – an *acquired* taste. It's extremely tart and fizzy; in fact, we always say of ours that if it doesn't make the hairs on the back of your neck stand up, it's not doing its job!

On the farm we're all used to the taste by now, and even my son, Benji, can drink it straight up. You can sweeten your kefir by blending it with fruit, but if you do that, be sure to consume it immediately. Don't let it sit overnight, as the fructose (fruit sugar) will degrade the power of the probiotics.

If you need some extra persuasion to get kefir down the necks of your more resistant family members, you can try these tried-and-tested kefir smoothie recipes. You could also get hold of an inexpensive ice-lolly maker, and freeze the smoothies to make kefir ice lollies. They won't know it's healthy until it's too late!

### *Benji's Special*

170 ml (6 fl oz) kefir

1 banana

Half an avocado

1 tbsp cold-pressed virgin flaxseed oil

Stevia, to taste

**Note**: depending on the type of stevia you use, start with a pinch and work up gradually – stevia is many times sweeter than sugar).

Put the ingredients in a blender and blitz until smooth. This is the classic kefir smoothie, and our little boy's favorite. It's great for kids, and for grown-ups who like it sweet! The avocado makes it creamy without disturbing the taste, and adds those good fats that you need to heal the skin (more on these later).

## Strawberry Surprise

170 ml (6 fl oz) kefir

A handful of frozen or fresh strawberries

½ tsp pure vanilla extract

1 tbsp cold-pressed virgin flaxseed oil

Stevia, to taste

Put the ingredients in a blender and blitz until smooth. Easy on the eyes, and the tastebuds, this one is pretty in pink. If you prefer, you can substitute raspberries or forest fruits for the strawberries.

## Blueberry Super Smoothie

170 ml (6 fl oz) kefir

A handful of fresh or frozen blueberries

1 tbsp maca powder

1 tbsp cold-pressed virgin flaxseed oil

Stevia, to taste

Put the ingredients in a blender and blitz until smooth. The malty-tasting maca powder gives this lovely purple superfood drink a kick.

## Virgin Pina Colada

170 ml (6 fl oz) kefir

1 banana

1 tbsp virgin coconut oil

Stevia, to taste

Add two chunks of pineapple, if desired.

Put the ingredients in a blender and blitz until smooth. A delicious tropical treat – close your eyes and pretend you're on a sunny beach!

## Bounty Bar

170 ml (6 fl oz) kefir

1 tbsp raw cocoa powder

1 tbsp coconut oil

Stevia, to taste

Put the ingredients in a blender and blitz until smooth. This healthy version of the classic candy bar is great for staving off those late-afternoon sweet-treat cravings.

### �֍ GSS TAKEAWAYS ✖

◈ Drinking kefir will re-populate your microbiome; if you don't see significant improvement in your skin condition after your first 21-day 'course,' try another.

◈ Three back-to-back courses of kefir are generally effective for all but the most severe skin conditions.

◈ Kefir is lactose-free.

◈ You can blend kefir with fruit and stevia to make it more palatable, or make smoothies with it.

◈ If you make kefir at home, you should ferment it until the pH is below 4.5 and test your kefir regularly at a public health laboratory to ensure that your grains have not acquired a bacteriophage infection.

Chapter 15

# GSS Habit #2: Use Goat's Milk Kefir Skincare

While you're taking your course(s) of kefir, use goat's milk-based kefir skincare in place of your usual cleanser and moisturizer. Wash your skin with a kefir cleanser and apply a lotion containing kefir twice daily, to all affected areas.

Using probiotic skincare products containing kefir will put the good bugs back into your skin biome, and restore balance to the microbial community there.

Once your skin condition has cleared, you can continue using kefir-based skincare indefinitely. It will act as a natural skin shield, keeping the skin microbiome primed with beneficial bacteria that will prevent future flare-ups.

## Applying kefir skincare

You can either buy kefir-based cleansers and lotions (*see Resource section*) or apply your homemade kefir directly to your skin. The latter process is not particularly easy or convenient (as I discovered when I applied it directly to Rich's skin!), which is part of the reason I developed a kefir skincare range. But you can simply pat the kefir directly onto the skin with a flannel, allow it to dry for 30 minutes, then rinse off.

It's safe to apply kefir skincare directly to inflamed skin, but avoid applying it to broken skin, as the lactic acid in the kefir (a gentle exfoliant that aids skin cell renewal) may cause stinging. Kefir can also be poured into your bath water, to give your skin a boost of healing beneficial bacteria.

It's important that the kefir in the skincare you choose is made with goat's milk rather than cow's, as goat's milk possesses the unique ability to penetrate the barrier of the human skin, carrying a valuable cargo of anti-inflammatories, vitamins, and minerals.

## Ditch the chemicals

Environmental toxins such as parabens, phthalates, petrochemicals, dyes, and perfumes are often found in personal care products and will damage your microbiome, so it's important to get rid of anything you're currently using that contains these nasties.

Research has found that the average woman 'hosts' around 515 unique chemicals by the time she finishes her grooming and make-up routine in the morning. These chemicals can leach into the system and alter our DNA.[1] The cells then fail to recognize one another, and fire on each other. This 'friendly fire' is the definition of *auto* (meaning *self*) immune; it literally causes your system to attack itself.[2]

So while you're following the GSS, do a clean sweep of your bathroom cabinet. Purge your personal care routine of anything that contains harmful chemicals that you can't pronounce!

For more guidance on natural alternatives, I recommend Janey Lee Grace's book *Look Great Naturally... Without Ditching the Lipstick* (Hay House, 2013).

## Coming off steroids

For those of you who've been using steroid creams on your (or your child's) eczema for longer than four weeks, it's important that you begin the 'tapering-off' process immediately, reducing usage to twice weekly (steroids should never be abruptly stopped) and then eventually weaning yourself off them completely.

The UK's National Eczema Association has issued the following urgent education announcement on the home page of its website regarding the use of topical corticosteroids (TCS):

*Do not use daily TCS continuously for more than two to four weeks – then the frequency should be tapered to twice weekly use. Your provider should strive to help create a safe and effective long-term treatment plan that does not include daily use of TCS, especially on more sensitive areas.*

*Close follow up and careful monitoring with good communication will help ensure this. Do not ask for multiple refills without evaluation, or questioning the usage pattern.[3]*

## *Why the urgency?*

The danger of prolonged, frequent, or overuse of moderate to high-potency TCS is an adverse effect known as topical steroid withdrawal syndrome, sometimes called topical steroid addiction or Red Skin Syndrome.

Basically, your skin becomes addicted to the steroid creams, and the results can be horrific. If you want to frighten yourself, consider the story of Janelle Norman, who went through this process and describes her experience in this way:

'My skin was becoming so inflamed, it was starting to crack. It was starting to burn more and more, and the symptoms just got stronger and stronger. Eventually my skin started to split, and it started to ooze and crack off. There was so much blood, so much pain, and my hair started to fall out. I was just in pure misery. I could not sleep; I could barely eat.'[4]

The Topical Steroid Awareness Network (ITSAN.org) has been founded to help people like Janelle.

**Long story short:** *steroid creams are not a long-term solution for eczema.* **The only answer is to provide your microbiome with the good bugs it needs to function properly.**

## How topical probiotics help the skin

Probiotic kefir-based skincare may be used for treatment of eczema in place of steroids. You can begin to use it immediately and continue through the process of weaning yourself off steroids. Kefir skincare will not harm your skin in any way. The probiotics it contains will become more effective once you stop using the steroids altogether.

In fact, emerging dermatological research is indicating a link between the use of topical probiotics – in the form of lotions and cleansers – and clearer skin in acne and rosacea patients too. According to US dermatology expert Whitney P. Bowe, there are three ways that probiotic bacteria are useful when applied topically:

1. **As a protective shield.** In acne and rosacea patients, microorganisms on the skin are recognized as foreign by the body's immune system, which springs into action to deal with this potential threat. The result? Inflammation, and the redness or bumps common in these autoimmune-related skin conditions.

   Probiotics applied topically in a soap or cream sit on the skin's surface and prevent the skin cells from 'seeing' the microbes that can cause an immune system response. This is known as 'bacterial interference,' as probiotics protect the skin and interfere with the ability of bad bugs, bacteria, or parasites to provoke an immune reaction.

2. **Antimicrobial properties.** Sometimes the substances produced by probiotics have antimicrobial properties, which enables them to create holes in bad bacteria and kill them. In much the same way that antibiotics work in the treatment of acne and rosacea, probiotics can help prevent harmful bugs from triggering skin inflammation.

3. **A calming effect.** When certain types of probiotics are placed in contact with skin cells, they calm the parts of the cells that may want to react to the presence of bad bacteria seen as a threat. These healthy signals produced by the probiotics stop the skin cells from sending the 'attack'

messages to the immune system that result in flares of acne or rosacea.[5]

## ✿ GSS TAKEAWAYS ✿

⊕ Use goat's milk kefir-based skincare while you're following the GSS, and beyond, for the sake of your microbiome.

⊕ The average woman 'hosts' 515 unique chemicals during her bathroom routine. These can leach into our bodies, alter our DNA and cause autoimmune disorders.

⊕ If you've been using steroids for eczema or psoriasis for longer than four weeks, it's vital that you begin the tapering-off process immediately, to avoid topical steroid withdrawal.

⊕ Instead of steroids and harsh, chemical-based personal care products, use gentle, natural, probiotic skincare. This will re-populate the beneficial bacteria on your skin biome.

⊕ Early research suggests that topical probiotics – in the form of lotions and cleansers – can benefit those with acne and rosacea.

Chapter 16

# GSS Habit #3:
# Drink Bone Broth

During your course(s) of kefir, drink at least one mug of warm bone broth every day. Once your skin condition has improved, you can continue drinking bone broth for the rest of your life!

Bone broth is an easy, inexpensive way to get bio-available collagen into your system. Collagen is the holy grail of beauty – and an important part of the GSS because it's the 'glue' of the body, giving our skin strength and elasticity, and helping to replace dead skin cells. Our bodies stop producing collagen as we age, so it becomes increasingly important over time.

You can have more than one mug of broth daily if you wish, and you can drink them at a time that works for you. I like to drink mine first thing in the morning, even before having my kefir! But it's also lovely as a late afternoon pick-me-up.

## Bone broth + kefir = gut healing

Bone broth works beautifully in tandem with kefir. The idea behind this two-step healing process is to:

1.  Heal the lining of the gut with bone broth.

2.  Re-populate the newly healed gut with the good bugs in the kefir.

The lining of your gut is only one cell thick, and it's under constant assault from the antibiotics and chemicals in your environment. These can cause tiny tears or 'leaks' in the gut lining, allowing improperly broken-down food molecules to escape into your bloodstream, where they wreak havoc on your immune system.

Drinking bone broth and kefir provides a continuous healing, soothing action that repairs your gut, and then keeps it in good repair and prevents further damage.

How will you know that your gut is healed? When your skin is clear, your digestion is smooth and pain-free, and your energy levels are high! By the time you're feeling this good, my guess is that you'll be committed to carrying on with both the broth and the kefir. After all, why would you ever stop such nourishing, beneficial habits?

## The magic of bone broth

I discovered bone broth in the same way I have most things – by accident, out of necessity. On the farm we keep many meat animals. Rich does his own butchering, and we end up with large amounts of meat in the chest freezer. In my early days as a farmer's wife, I was baffled by these big frozen lumps of bone-in meat – they were too hard to cut, and too big to sauté. What was I supposed to do with them?

'Make cawl,' Rich advised. At the time, I'd never heard of cawl, but I soon discovered that it's a traditional Welsh meat stew. The idea is to simmer a meat carcass – bones with meat still attached – for at least two hours, to make the base of the cawl. Sometimes I used meat that was left over from a Sunday roast; it's a thrifty way to get every bit of value from our food.

Alternately, when we butcher a lamb on the farm, we put aside the cuts that are too poor or gristly for roasting, and bag and freeze them, ready to make cawl. Once the meaty bones have been simmered, they are removed and the cooked meat is picked off. It's then put back into the pot, along with vegetables. This makes for a delicious, hearty supper.

By the time I read *The Bone Broth Secret: A Culinary Adventure in Health, Beauty, Longevity* by Louise Hay and Heather Dane, I'd already been making bone broth (in the form of cawl) for ages without knowing it. (I heartily recommend this book by the way; it's fun, easy to read, and full of both good science and great recipes.)

These days I nearly always have a large pot of bone broth simmering away in the farmhouse kitchen. Once I understood the power of bone broth, I became a dedicated fan and advocate. I sip a mug of warm broth first thing in the morning, with a bit of sea salt and lemon. It's soothing, nourishing, filling, and gets my day off to a great start.

The secret of bone broth is reflected in its name – it's stock that's made with *bones*. Our ancestors cooked with bones – they wasted nothing! They ate the meat, then turned the scraps and bones into nourishing stews. These days, of course, we buy everything by weight, from the supermarket, so it's rare to find meat with the bones still in it. And if we do have something with bones, like a chicken carcass, we tend to discard them.

## The power of collagen

Bone broth's magic lies in the fact that cooking down the tendons, joints, and ligaments in the meat bones denatures collagen into an easily digestible form called gelatin. Gelatin protects the intestines by lining the mucous membrane and helping to heal the gut. This can help resolve digestive problems, which is why bone broth is recommended by Dr. Natasha Campbell McBride in her GAPS (Gut and Psychology Syndrome) Diet.

**Your body needs collagen to maintain glowing skin, hair, and nails. It also serves to support, strengthen, provide structure and hold the body together.**

And after age 40, your body no longer produces collagen. So a mug of bone broth every day will put this amazing stuff back into your body, where it can achieve powerful results.

## Making bone broth

The following recipe, which serves four, will give you a delicious Welsh cawl to serve for supper, and also a supply of bone broth for you to re-heat and drink as part of the GSS.

## Bone broth (followed by Welsh Cawl)

1 chicken carcass (including leftover meat and bones). Beef or lamb will also work, but I find pork a bit too greasy.

2 tsp sea salt

5 whole black peppercorns

8 carrots

16 new potatoes

1 onion

1 swede

1 leek

### Instructions for the bone broth

1.  If you have a roast on a Sunday, just throw all the bones from the main carcass into a big *saucepan. If you're starting from scratch, roast a whole chicken (or lamb or beef joint), then remove the meat (which can be used for another dish) and put the carcass into the pan. For both methods, add water until it's about 5 cm (2 inches) from the top of the pan.

    * The saucepan I use is a whopping 20 litres (5 gallons), but then I have a big family. Still, bone broth is such a brilliant thing that I'm going to encourage you to make extra and freeze a lot of it – so a large 10-litre (2.5-gallon) pan is a good thing to buy.

2.  Bring to the boil, then lower the heat to a simmer. Leave to cook for at least two–three hours, more if you can (the longer the better; our bone broth simmers all day). The magic is bones+water+time. If you're at work during the day, treat yourself to a slow cooker, and simmer your

broth all day in that. Just put in enough water to ensure it doesn't go dry. The smell will uplift you when you come through the door at the end of the day, and give you the strength to put together the rest of the supper!

3. Once the broth has been cooking for a sufficient length of time, sieve out the bones and meat by tipping the broth into another pan with a large colander sitting in it.

4. Pour about half the broth into a separate container, let it cool thoroughly, and then store it in the fridge for up to three days. For the next three mornings, you can ladle broth into a mug and heat it up; try it with a bit of sea salt and a squeeze of lemon.

5. If you've more bone broth than you can get through in three days (don't keep it in the fridge longer than that, as it's the perfect environment for bad bacteria), you can freeze it in large silicon ice-cube trays, made for freezing baby food, and pop out one at a time to thaw and re-heat.

Always re-heat bone broth in a saucepan, never in a microwave – it's just as fast. The microwave distorts the molecules in your food, which is a bad idea when you're trying to improve your health! We don't have a microwave on the farm... and we don't miss it. I find re-heating my homemade leftovers is easily done on the stovetop or in the oven.

## Instructions for the Welsh cawl

1. Put the remaining broth back onto the heat and continue simmering. Place the meat and bones (now sitting in the colander) to one side to allow the whole thing to cool.

2. Add the vegetables to the pan. I use those listed above, but you can try whatever your family likes. They can all be chopped quite roughly, in big pieces – this is a hearty peasant-style stew. Simmer the vegetables in the broth for about an hour.

3. Once the meat and bones in the colander have cooled enough to handle comfortably, pick any remaining meat off the bones. It should now come away easily. Add the meat back into the pot 15 minutes before serving.

   **Note**: you can re-use bones for broth at least twice before discarding them – just pop them into the freezer until you're ready to make cawl again.

4. You now have a delicious cawl for supper! To give it a traditional Welsh feel, chop up a leek and toss it in, along with the cooled meat, 15 minutes before you're ready to serve. Season to taste with more sea salt and black pepper.

---

### ৯ GSS TAKEAWAYS ৯

- ⊕ Drinking bone broth puts bio-available collagen into your system.

- ⊕ Collagen is needed to heal the lining of the gut.

- ⊕ Bone broth and kefir work together to restore the health and proper function of the gut.

Chapter 17

# GSS Habit #4:
# Replace Sugar with Stevia

While you're following the GSS, there's one foodstuff you *really* need to let go of if you want to heal your skin condition: sugar. Why? Quite simply, sugar kills the good bugs in your microbiome.

Professor Cynthia Kenyon from the University of California, one of the world's top researchers in the field of aging, experimented with giving glucose to worms, and found that it shortened their life spans dramatically. She claims that if you could see what sugar does to living organisms, you would never eat sugar again. She doesn't.[1]

**Sugar is death to your microbiome. Just say 'no' to sugar.**

## A great sugar substitute

So what can you use as an alternative to sugar, something that's kinder to your skin and gut? I only allow one kind of sweetener on the farm: stevia. Stevia is brilliant stuff: it's made from the leaves of a plant, is low-GI, has zero calories, and is safe for diabetics. In fact, stevia is not actually a sweetener at all – it just stimulates the sweet tastebuds on your tongue, so you have the sensation of sweetness.

Stevia has been used for centuries as a bio-sweetener and a traditional treatment for diabetes – and studies show it may actually improve blood sugar control.[2] Stevia also appears to have anti-cancer, anti-inflammatory, antioxidant, and antibacterial properties.[3] Aside from diabetes, researchers particularly recommend its use for children, and for those wishing to lose weight.[4]

The sugar folks fought long and hard to keep stevia out of the UK and off the shelves – and who can blame them! You would too, if faced with an alternative to your product that had zero calories and actual health *benefits*.

The sugar barons lost the fight, though, and had to adopt a 'if you can't beat 'em, join 'em' approach, so stevia can now be found in many supermarkets.

**A word of advice:** carefully check the label on the stevia you find in the supermarket, because many brands have been layered onto a dextrose base to give the stevia extra bulk – and dextrose is a form of glucose (sugar) derived from starches.

## Ways to use stevia

I recommend using completely pure stevia, which comes in crystals, drops, and clickers that you can pop straight into coffee and tea. I usually order mine online, or get it from a health food store. Pure stevia is a bit expensive, but as it's roughly 30 times as sweet as sugar, one small bag will last for a long time.

The only downside to stevia that I've found is that it's hard to bake with. It has an odd, fluffy texture that can't match the lovely grainy quality that sugar gives a cake. If you find a good way to bake with it, please do let me know, and we'll go into business together!

There *is* a baking version of stevia that has erythritol added for bulk. Erythritol is a sugar alcohol that's made by fermenting glucose. Like stevia, it doesn't raise your blood sugar, so it is microbiome-safe. The advantages of erythritol is that it creates the same shiny effect in low-calorie chocolate, adds bulk to dairy products, and improves the shelf life of baked goods. Stevia and erythritol work for home baking because they're both heat-stable. It's safe enough, but I'm still not crazy about the results.

For baking, I prefer to sweeten with whole, blended-up fruit and veg, like bananas and carrots, or dried fruit. Dried fruit tends to have a similar glycemic index to its non-dried counterpart. So it's safe to use sparingly as a natural sweetener – because it still has its fiber, the sugar goes into your bloodstream more slowly.

Dried apples, apricots, peaches, and plums are all low GI and nice to work with. If you need to increase sweetness levels, you can top up with stevia until it's sweet enough for your taste.

**Important note:** Pregnant or nursing women shouldn't use stevia. Whole stevia leaves were traditionally used as a contraceptive by the Guarani Indians in Paraguay. Those on blood pressure or diabetes medications should check with their doctor before using stevia-based products, as they may interact with these medications. People allergic to ragweed may be allergic to stevia as well.

## What about other natural sweeteners?

You may be wondering about the effect of other natural and artificial sweeteners on the microbiome. Let's look at a few of the key ones now.

### Honey

Honey is brilliant stuff, but I use it only as a medicine. It's very high on the glycemic index – almost as high as pure glucose – so don't use it as an everyday sweetener as it will damage your microbiome. (See habit #6 for more on the glycemic index.)

Honey is a natural antibiotic. On the farm, if we have coughs or colds, we make a mix of honey, lemon, and ginger and drink it down. We also apply sterile dressings that have been surgically infused with honey to wounds, in order to promote rapid healing and prevent infection. I used these surgical honey dressings on Rich's wound when he had MRSA, and I always keep a few spare in my farmhouse first-aid kit.[5]

**Note:** Honey should not be mixed with kefir, though, because its naturally antibiotic action will kill off the probiotics that you're trying to get into your system.

We don't bother with manuka honey – apparently, three times more manuka honey is on the shelves than is actually produced in New Zealand, so the chances are, you're being overcharged for fake manuka.[6]

When we need medical honey on the farm, we use heather honey – the type that most beekeepers choose to eat. It's a little more expensive than regular honey, but nowhere near as pricey as manuka! It's a mono-honey (made from only one plant) that's been shown to be just as anti-bacterially effective as manuka.[7] It's a UK-made product too, which is something we like to support.

## Maple and agave syrup

I don't use these as daily sweeteners, although I do treat myself to real maple syrup on pancakes for special occasions. Maple syrup is even higher on the glycemic index than honey, so it's not good for your microbiome either.

And *please* don't use agave syrup while you are following the GSS! Agave nectar is about 85 percent fructose, which is *much higher* than plain sugar, and can contribute to insulin resistance when consumed in large amounts.

## Artificial sweeteners

I don't approve of these, so we don't use them on the farm. I do chew xylitol gum, though, because it's been shown to promote dental health. But stevia is the only thing that goes onto my farmhouse kitchen table, or into my NutriBullet to mix with my kefir.

## ✿ GSS TAKEAWAYS ✿

✦ Pure stevia is a safe, natural sweetener that, unlike refined sugar, doesn't harm the microbiome.

✦ Honey has natural antibiotics that impair the action of probiotics, so it's not an appropriate sweetener for kefir.

✦ Agave syrup and maple syrup are both high-GI sweeteners that can harm the microbiome.

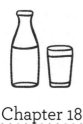

## Chapter 18

# GSS Habit #5:
# Eat Goat Dairy

While following the GSS, choose dairy products made from goat's milk, rather than cow's milk.

In many parts of the world, goat's milk is preferred to cow's milk. However, in the West, we tend to favor cow dairy, which is a shame, because goat's milk is nutritious, healthy, and fabulous for both our skin and our gut.

In fact, after conducting a study into the nutritional characteristics of goat's milk, a group of scientists at the Department of Physiology at the University of Granada in Spain declared it a 'natural functional food'[1] (functional foods are those that deliver additional or enhanced health benefits beyond their basic nutritional value).

## Goat's milk vs cow's milk

Below are some very good reasons why those with eczema, psoriasis, acne, or rosacea should add goat's milk products to their diet – and drop the cow's milk.

### Seven reasons to go for goat

1. **Cow dairy is incredibly allergenic for human beings.** It's mucous-producing, and a known trigger for eczema. According to cowsmilkallergy.co.uk, up to 1 in 20 British children under the age of three are allergic to cow's milk. Symptoms of cow's milk allergy, or CMA, include the following (especially if accompanied by restless sleep or excessive crying):

- Eczema

- Diarrhea

- Colic

- Constipation

- Wheezing

- Vomiting/reflux

And it's not just the kids who suffer. Recent research has shown that more adults than previously believed suffer from CMA, although they've usually blamed their symptoms on lactose intolerance.[2]

Cow's milk contains casein alpha 1 – a protein found in mammalian milk that's been identified as an allergen. Goat's milk contains less casein alpha 1 than cow's milk, so goat's milk is considered hypoallergenic. The University of Granada researchers pointed out that 'For this reason, in some countries [goat's milk] is used as the basis for the development of infant formula in place of cow milk.'[3]

2. **Goat's milk may be better for our health than cow's milk**. The researchers at the University of Granada, in their comparative study on the properties of goat's and cow's milk, found that goat's milk has nutritional characteristics beneficial to health, largely because it has many nutrients that make it similar to human milk.

Their study found that goat's milk outperforms cow's milk in its ability to prevent ferropenic anaemia (iron deficiency) and bone demineralization (softening of the bones). It also helps with the digestive and metabolic utilization of minerals such as iron, calcium, phosphorus, and magnesium.[4]

3. **Goat's milk contains prebiotics, which feed probiotics.** Goat's milk has more oligosaccharides with a composition similar to that of human milk. These compounds reach the large intestine undigested and act as prebiotics (substances that make the pre-existing bugs in your gut healthier, so they can out-compete the bad bugs).[5]

4. **Goat's milk has a lower proportion of lactose than cow's milk.** As it's easier to digest, many people with intolerance to this milk sugar can tolerate goat's milk.[6]

5. **Goat's milk has smaller fat molecules than cow's milk, and a healthier type of fat.** Goat's milk contains more essential omega-6 fatty acids (linoleic and archidonic) than cow's milk.

Goat's milk also has 30–35 percent medium-chain fatty acids, while cow's milk only has 15–20 percent. These fatty acids are a quick source of energy and are not stored as body fat.[7]

6. **Goat's milk can lower cholesterol.** Goat's milk fat reduces total cholesterol levels and maintains adequate levels of triglycerides and transaminases (GOT and GPT). This makes it helpful for the prevention of heart disease.[8]

7. **Goat's milk helps with bone formation.** Goat's milk is rich in calcium and phosphorus in a bioavailable form, which helps with bone formation. It also has more zinc and selenium than cow's milk. These essential micronutrients also help prevent neurodegenerative diseases.[9]

Today it's easy to find goat's milk, cheese, butter, and yogurt in any quality supermarket. So switch to goat dairy, and remove cow dairy from your diet for good.

---

### ⚘ GSS TAKEAWAYS ⚘

⊕ Scientist consider goat's milk a 'functional food,' with health benefits for humans.

⊕ Cow's milk is allergenic and a common trigger for eczema and asthma.

⊕ Goat's milk has less lactose and smaller fat globules than cow's milk, which makes it more easily tolerated by those with allergy or intolerance to the latter.

Chapter 19

# GSS Habit #6:
# Choose Slow-Burning Foods

The GSS is about eating to support the health of your gut. As part of this, it's important to add more foods with a low glycemic index (GI) to your diet. These foods 'burn' more slowly in your digestive system, releasing their nutrients gradually over time.

The glycemic index (GI) is a number value assigned to carbohydrate-containing foods based on how slowly or quickly those foods cause increases in blood sugar levels. Low-GI foods, among them oatmeal, barley, lentils, and chickpeas, take a long time to break down in your system, and are better for your skin than high-GI foods like bread, rice, white potatoes, and processed foods. High-GI foods burn very quickly inside your body, creating a rush of insulin that upsets your system and sets up a pattern of craving.

Remember, your skin is just a map of your gut. So if you de-stabilize your microbiome with high-GI foods, the results will show up on your skin.

You want to eat things that will slowly trickle blood sugar into your system, keeping your microbiome platform steady and secure. And avoid things that wobble it, causing general panic and upheaval inside your system! Your skin will thank you.

## Sugar doesn't always taste sweet

As we've already discovered, too much sugar kills off the good bugs in your microbiome. But that means too much systemic blood sugar as well, not just the white refined stuff.

As far as your microbiome's concerned, *sugar isn't just the stuff that tastes sweet.* Everything you eat is eventually broken down into blood sugar (glucose), and that's what fuels your cells.

**So the important question is not, 'Does this food taste sweet?' It's 'How fast is my body turning this food into sugar?' The answer should be: 'Slowly!'**

Let's take a closer look at this process. Your entire system – all of the magic bugs that make up your body, along with your muscles, your brain, your heart, and your liver, which drive all of the trillions of cascading actions that occur every second of the day – needs energy to work, and this energy comes from the food you eat.

The bugs in your gut digest your food by mixing it with fluids from your stomach. During this process, the sugar and starches in the food are broken down into blood sugar (glucose). The bugs in your stomach and gut absorb the glucose, and then re-release it into your bloodstream. Once there, glucose can be used immediately for energy or stored for later use.

But glucose alone is not enough to fuel your system. You also need insulin – a hormone produced in the pancreas that regulates the amount of glucose in the blood. Insulin is necessary for your body to use or store glucose for energy. Without it, glucose just loiters around uselessly in the bloodstream.

So clever, hard-working little cells called beta cells run a constant monitoring system on the amount of glucose in your bloodstream. They check your glucose level every few seconds, and sense when they need to speed up or slow down the amount of insulin they're making and releasing. Understand, these poor little guys are just trying to keep everything stable. And usually, we don't make it very easy for them.

## The glycemic index

Different foods do different things to our glucose levels. And much of the food we eat these days dumps huge amounts of blood sugar into our system, all at once.

The glycemic index (GI) gives us an idea of how fast our body converts the carbohydrates in a food into glucose. Two foods with the same amount of carbohydrate can have different GI values. If a food has a low GI value, it means that it raises glucose levels only a little bit. A high GI value means that it raises them a lot, all at once.

To get a sense of the impact this has on your microbiome, imagine that you're making a fire in the fireplace, using only newspaper. It will flare up with a huge, bright *whoooosh* – and then fade right down before burning out.

That's what happens inside your system when you eat something that is 'high GI.' The glucose level in the blood soars, and the beta cells trigger the pancreas to release a lot more insulin into the bloodstream, to deal with all the blood sugar.

The excess insulin in your system then causes you to crave more sugar. So you eat more sugar, the beta cells dump in more insulin – and after enough repeated cycles like this, you can end up with type 2 diabetes. Basically, you've exhausted your body's insulin system by causing repeated blood sugar spikes.

But here's the kicker:

It's *not just things that taste sweet that create this cycle*. It's also anything that raises your glucose level rapidly, including everyday foods such as bread, potatoes, and rice.

Your body burns these up quickly, like newspaper in the fireplace.

In order to function well, your microbiome needs to be in 'homeostasis,' which is 'maintaining a constant internal environment.' This is what your hard-working system is trying to do. Dump a load of sugar in there, cause a quick, brief 'paper' fire that flares and then abruptly dies down, and there's no way to maintain a steady environment.

## GI values of common foods

The glycemic index compares everything to pure glucose, which has a rating of 100. Any food with a GI value over 70 is considered high; 56–69 is medium; and 55 or less is low. This chart shows the GI values of some everyday foods.

| Food | Glycemic index (glucose = 100) |
|---|---|
| White rice | 83 |
| Brown rice | 66 |
| White bread | 71 |
| Whole wheat bread | 71 |
| Pasta (white spaghetti) | 44 |
| White potato (boiled) | 82 |
| Sweet potato (boiled) | 46 |
| New potato (boiled) | 62 |
| Ice cream | 57 |
| Lentils | 29 |
| Chickpeas | 10 |
| Hummus (chickpea dip) | 6 |
| Oatmeal (rough cut) | 55 |

Sorry to be the bearer of bad news here, but as you can see, white potatoes turn to sugar in your system faster than ice cream. And because the insulin spike that produces damages your microbiome, you're going to see the results on your skin.

It's the same for bread – both white and whole wheat. There's almost no difference in the rate that your body burns these two foodstuffs. Ditto for white rice and brown rice. If you presume that brown is always better than white, you may be surprised to find that, often, there's little difference in the speed at which they are converted to sugar.

# Go low GI to help your microbiome

So, if eating bread, rice, and potatoes is like burning newspaper in our system, causing an abrupt rush of glucose and de-stabilizing our microbiome, what *can* we eat to support our microbiome health? The answer is – a diet rich in slow-burning foods.

We want to build our fire with wood, not newspaper. We want to eat things that will burn slowly inside our system, and keeping it ticking over.

**This GSS habit is so important!** To keep your microbiome healthy and your skin clear, you must eat low-GI foods and avoid high-GI ones. This is not a fad diet, but a long-term change to your eating habits that will sustain you over a lifetime. You'll find that it also has great benefits for weight loss, energy, and digestion.

## *What are slow-burning foods?*

So what are the winners in the slow-burner sweepstakes? Think oatmeal. Think pulses, amaranth, millet, or quinoa. Anything you have to chew a lot! Think healthy fats (coming up in the next chapter). Protein is good. Fruit and veg are good. Pasta – surprisingly – is pretty low GI. (It has to do with the physical organization of the starch granules in the pasta dough.) But cook pasta al dente, and don't have it too often.

If you love potatoes, choose sweet potatoes, which oddly have a score of just 46. (Note that it's better to boil sweet potatoes rather than baking them, which raises their GI.) New potatoes sneak into the GI score table at 62, which still beats a boiled white potato at 82.

One high GI food that we think of as healthy is fruit juice. Commercial juices – with the fruit pulp removed – burn in your system quickly. So don't juice your fruit – blend it! Whizz up a whole piece of fruit in the blender and drink it with the pulp included; it will burn inside your system much more slowly.

Carbohydrates that are digested slowly and therefore don't produce high spikes in glucose levels are good; these include whole grains, legumes and pulses (beans, lentils, and chickpeas) and other high-fiber foods. An added bonus is that a diet rich in these low-GI foods reduces the markers of inflammation associated with chronic disease, including cancer and heart disease.[1]

## A word about gluten

Gluten is an elastic protein formed when moisture is added to flour. Commonly found in wheat, rye, and barley, it's a kind of glue that holds the proteins in grains together. It's not just found in bread, but also in pizza dough, cereals, soups, and sauces.

Although a relatively small percentage of the population have celiac disease – a serious illness in which the body's immune system attacks itself when gluten is eaten – a lot of people are sensitive to gluten. Because it's an allergen, the presence of gluten can trigger the immune system, which produces the symptoms of allergy and inflammation, including acne, eczema, psoriasis and rosacea.

So we suggest that while on the GSS, you avoid gluten as much as possible. Instead, try alternative grains like millet, amaranth, teff, and quinoa.

These have the advantage of being both non-allergenic and low-GI – so get out of your wheat rut, and ditch the gluten.

## ❧ GSS TAKEAWAYS ❧

❖ A diet rich in slow-digesting, low-GI foods can help your skin and gut, and protect against disease.

❖ The GI rating of a food is an indicator of how rapidly your system turns it into sugar.

❖ High GI foods burn quickly, while low GI foods burn slowly. Fast-burners de-stabilize your microbiome, while slow-burners keep it stable.

❖ Avoid gluten-containing grains like wheat, which can cause inflammation. Go for gluten-free, low-GI grains like millet, amaranth, teff, and quinoa.

Chapter 20

# GSS Habit #7: Go for Good Fats

We've been taught to fear and avoid *all* fats, but it turns out those naysayers were wrong. Some fats are good for you! And you won't be able to heal your skin without adding them to your diet.

Here on the farm, we're big fans of both good fats and natural goat dairy products. And goat's butter is both! That's right: eaten in moderation, butter made from goat's milk is good for you. Here's why…

## Choose butter for butyrate

Butter provides naturally occurring butyrate to our diet. Butyrate is a short-chain fatty acid that boosts our immune system and reduces inflammation. **Anything that contains butyrate may also enhance intestinal barrier function and improve overall gut health.** (Side note: cow's butter also contains butyrate, but the GSS cautions against cow's dairy because of its allergenic properties.)

Goat's butter is much better for us than margarine, which contains trans fats: industrially produced nasties that have now been associated with a greater risk of coronary heart disease and early death. A recent study has found that butter, on the other hand, is not associated with an increased risk of death, heart disease, stroke, or type 2 diabetes.[1]

## A reduction in cholesterol

If you're worried about raising your cholesterol, don't be. A recent study showed that butter actually leads to less elevation of blood fats after a meal, even when compared with olive oil.[2]

Why is this the case? About 20 percent of the fat in butter consists of short and medium-length fatty acids, which are 'good' fatty acids. These are used directly by the body as energy and so don't really affect our blood fat levels very much.

Scientists have long puzzled over 'the French paradox,' which is: how come those French folks have low cardiovascular disease rates, despite a delicious diet high in saturated fats? Well, the answer may lie in a staple French food: cheese.

Recent research found that study participants who consumed cheese had higher fecal levels of butyrate, that magical compound produced by happy gut bacteria. And here's the best bit: elevated butyrate levels were linked to a reduction in cholesterol.[3]

So feed your good bugs goat's butter and cheese! This stuff makes your immune system sing. Improved immune function means improved gut health, which will help to clear your skin.

Having said that, do be reasonable! Over-consumption of anything will eventually cause problems, so enjoy your food – and your fats – in moderate amounts.

## More 'good' fats

Besides goat's butter and cheese, it's important to add other good fats into your daily diet. Choose monounsaturated and polyunsaturated fats such as olive oil, avocado, walnuts (and other nuts), seeds, and oily fish (salmon, mackerel, sardines).

### Eggs

On the farm, we eat a lot of egg scrambles. Eggs are a great source of protein, lipids, vitamins, and minerals, and contain as many disease-busting antioxidants as apples do.[4] Dr. Natasha Campbell McBride, author of *Gut and Psychology Syndrome* and founder of the GAPS diet, recommends eggs, saying: 'Eggs are one of the most nourishing and easy to digest foods on this planet.'

Eggs are a perfect base for carrying other healthy fats: I love tossing half an avocado, some salmon and cubes of goat's cheese into a skillet with two eggs for a super-quick and healthy lunch.

### Flaxseed oil

Flaxseed oil is another great addition to the diet: it's an amazing source of healthy omega-3 fatty acids. In the Budwig Diet Protocol,[5] Dr. Josh Axe recommends combining flaxseed oil with kefir. This is based on the groundbreaking work of

Dr. Joanna Budwig, historically one of the world's leading authorities on fats and oils.

An easy way to get this healthy combo into your daily routine is to simply blend one tablespoon of cold-pressed virgin flaxseed oil into your daily kefir smoothie (*see the smoothie recipes in habit #1*). Flaxseed oil is fragile, so be sure to keep it in the fridge and observe 'best before' dates.

## Coconut oil

This is another good fat that should definitely be a GSS regular. Scientists say that coconut oil is one of the few foods that actually deserves the title 'superfood.' Its unique combination of fatty acids can have a profound positive effect on health, including fat loss, better brain function, and many other benefits.[6]

Coconut oil has been shown to control overgrowth of candida albicans in mice,[7] and the lauric acid in coconut kills acne bacteria.[8] It has also been shown to be a safe and effective moisturizer for dry skin, with natural antiseptic effects.[9]

Personally, I don't cook with coconut oil, as I don't really want everything tasting of coconut. But one tablespoon blended into a kefir smoothie works beautifully; or just put a spoonful straight into your mouth. Allow it to dissolve and then swallow, and you'll also reap the oil-pulling benefits for your teeth and gums – coconut oil's natural antibiotic action attacks the bacteria that cause tooth decay.[10]

## Avocados

These days, everyone's talking about how great avocados are, and I'm happy to add my voice to the choir. Avocados are high in oleic acid, which is an omega 9 fat that maintains moisture in the epidermal layer of the skin, helping to keep it soft and hydrated. Oleic acid also helps regenerate damaged skin cells and reduces facial redness and irritation,[11] making avocados an essential element of the GSS.

Avocados are also a great natural appetite suppressant, so if you're trying to shift a bit of excess weight, throw half an avocado into a green smoothie and it will fill you up enough to call it supper.

## Walnuts

Walnuts are a handy GSS snack food. According to a recent scientific study, a diet rich in walnuts and walnut oil – sources of polyunsaturated omega 3 fatty acids – could help our bodies better respond to stress, and reduce bad cholesterol and inflammation.[12] We keep a bowl of walnuts on the farmhouse table to grab throughout the day – I find if I make it easy for the boys, they're more likely to go for the healthy option!

### ❊ GSS TAKEAWAYS ❊

✦ Regular consumption of the 'good' fats found in foods such as avocados, nuts, seeds, oily fish, olive oil, and flaxseed oil will improve the health of your gut and therefore your skin.

✦ Butter is a source of butyrate, which boosts the immune system and maintains healthy gut barrier function.

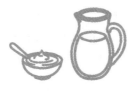

Conclusion

# Three Essential Lessons

Being in contact with the natural world on the farm has taught me more than I could ever have learned from books. Along the way, I've discovered three essential lessons, and I'd like to share these with you before you go on your way.

1. Get outside!

2. Nature has the answers.

3. We're all interconnected.

## Get outside!

As a city girl, I had an inborn resistance to getting wet, dirty, and muddy. The farm has certainly cured me of that – and taught me how valuable and important it is to spend some time outside every day, no matter what the weather.

That first breath of fresh air in the morning strengthens and refreshes me, and makes me remember exactly what our daily struggle is all about. When our lives are full of stress, getting outside into nature is a great way to boost our immune system and improve our skin in the process. Here's why...

## Walking in nature makes us healthier

Science has shown that walking in general is good for us, but walking in the woods, in a park, or any other green space, is even better at reducing stress and improving our physical and mental health.

According to Dr. Aaron Michelfelder, professor of family medicine at Loyola University Chicago Stritch School of Medicine in the US, going for a walk after a stressful day helps us wind down and reconnect.

'Our stress hormones [cortisol] rise all day long in our bloodstream,' he says. 'Taking even a few moments while walking to reconnect with your inner thoughts, and to check in with your body, will lower those damaging stress hormones. Walking with our family or friends is also a great way to lower our blood pressure and make us happier.'[1]

Dr. Michelfelder has also drawn on research from Japan which shows that walking in nature boosts our immune system and may even play a role in fighting cancer. Plants emit a chemical called phytoncide that protects them from rotting and insects, and it's theorized that when people breathe in that chemical, there's an increase in the level of their 'natural killer' cells, which are part of a person's immune response to cancer.[2]

'When we walk in a forest or park,' Dr. Michelfelder says, 'our levels of white blood cells increase and it also lowers our pulse rate, blood pressure, and cortisol.'[3]

## Go talk to the animals!

Exposing your children to farm animals early in their lives can modify the mechanism of allergies, according to recent research from the University of Eastern Finland.[4] And, according to researchers from Aarhus University in Denmark, it's never too late to experience 'the farm effect' – even adults who move to farming areas, where they experience a wider range of environmental exposures than in cities, may see a considerable reduction in hypersensitivities and allergies.[5]

**The idea here is that your immune system *benefits from being challenged*.**

The immune systems of people who work in farming are often exposed to a wide range of bacteria, fungi, pollen, and other irritants that may trigger a response that protects them against hypersensitivity. Working in a farming environment may help to decrease hypersensitivity to the most widespread plant allergens: grass and birch pollen.[6]

Here's an interesting fact about allergies: avoiding triggers doesn't make things better. In fact, the more you expose yourself, the more the immune system is stimulated, and the less it will ultimately react to the trigger.[7] So *lean in* to those outdoor experiences, and give your immune system a good workout.

## Vitamin D can help eczema

Vitamin D – found naturally in sunlight – has been found to be helpful for eczema. A study involving 107 Mongolian children, all of whom had a history of eczema that worsened during the transition from autumn to winter, found that daily treatment with a vitamin D supplement significantly reduced their symptoms.

Eczema commonly gets worse during the winter, and scientists are now hypothesizing that it might be because sufferers get less Vitamin D from the sun during that time. The children in the Mongolian study who were treated with Vitamin D reported a 29 percent improvement.[8]

So if you have eczema, go outside and get some sunshine!

# Nature has the answers

When I needed to save my husband from an antibiotic-resistant superbug, I turned to nature and found the answers that I needed. Nature has never failed me yet.

**Nature provides the solutions to the problems that we humans have created for ourselves.**

We often insist on 'improving' on nature by boiling things down. We like to do things like extracting one active ingredient from a plant and putting it into pill form, so we can sell it and make money.

But our so-called 'cleverness' has ended up creating a lot of problems – resistant bacteria being one of them. And when we run out of options on the chemical road, nature is patiently waiting there to give us the answers to our self-created ills.

Why is this? I believe it's because nature works with *complexity*. Nature's tendency is not to simplify, but to *complexify*. This is because *complexity = resilience*. The more complex a system is, the more different choices of defense it has when it's attacked.

## We're all interconnected

On the farm, Rich mows the hay with his blue tractor. We feed the hay to the goats, and give them fresh bedding every day. Then we muck out their pens, and put all the muck onto a big compost heap. There, trillions of gorgeous little organisms immediately spring into action, doing their work, spinning the muck into 'black gold.'

Once the microbes have done their work in converting the muck into gorgeous sweet-smelling, crumbly stuff called *dom*, this natural fertilizer is spread on the hay fields, to make them grow again for the next season of mowing.

Our hay fields are ancient, and deep-rooted to bring the minerals up from far down in the earth. Because we don't use poisons on our fields, there are many different strains of meadow flowers blooming there, all of which nourish the goats. There are many different strains of bacteria in the muck, too, and they all help to cherish the strains of meadow flowers in the hay. It's a complex, rich natural system.

This microbial alchemy feeds the hay, the hay feeds the goats, the goat's milk feeds the kefir grains, the kefir feeds us, we feed the goats. We ride this wheel of transformation through the seasons, year after year.

## Microbes are our friends

This is as close to magic as I ever need to be. And the key to it all? Those tiny microbes in the compost heap and in the kefir vats. Just because you can't see them, doesn't mean they are unimportant! They are the star players, making it all go round. Without them, everything would collapse and die.

When we take visitors around the farm on open days, I always stop in front of our big compost heap, and I tell them: 'That big heap of dirty straw might not look like much, but it's actually the golden heart of our farm.'

Watching the microbes in the compost heap spin muck into rich fertilizer – and seeing the kefir grains transform milk into kefir – is where I learned the lesson of microbial diversity. And it's *just the same inside your gut*. You want a lot of diversity in there. A rich mix of living things. *More* life, not less. *Pro*biotics, not *anti*biotics.

## Make the right choices

And as it is outside, so it is inside you. *It's all the same thing.* We're a fractal – a pattern that repeats at every level, from the microbes inside us, to the world around us, to the stars above us. As humans, we've been given this astonishing gift.

We are the stewards both of our own internal microbiome and the external ecosystem around us. These are positions of power, and with power comes responsibility.

Your internal ecosystem is fragile, and complex, and beautiful. You hold ultimate dominion over what rains down on all those little critters in there, because you control the mouth of the holobiont. They're trying to interact with you, but ultimately you make the decisions, and you determine the weather.

The decisions you make affect all of your symbionts. They are counting on you to make the right choices – just as the animals in our care on the farm count on us to make the right choices regarding their welfare.

The principles are the same: in the outside environment and inside our microbiome:

1. Don't poison it.

2. Feed it what it needs, to keep it healthy.

3. Look after it with loving care.

4. Encourage diversity.

If we all do that, the planet will thrive – and we will, too. And that, surely, is good news!

## ✿ GSS TAKEAWAYS ✿

- Getting outside and walking in nature boosts your immune system.

- Vitamin D may help resolve eczema.

- Exposure to animals and the commensal bacteria found on farms, challenges our immune system, which lowers allergic reactions.

- Nature has the answers to problems that we humans have created with our chemical solutions.

- Antibiotics inhibit diversity; probiotics promote diversity.

- We're all interconnected.

- Become a good steward of your internal and external ecosystems.

# Let's Work Together!

You're on a journey, moving toward your own healing. Congratulations, and welcome! We're all on this journey together. I may not yet have had the privilege of meeting you face-to-face, but you and I are fellow pioneers in this brave endeavor.

We are linked – by the lovely Welsh word *perthyn* that my husband taught me when I moved to this country. It means 'belonging.'

So I made a special gift for you; it's a travel journal, to help track your progress. You can download this free 21-day GSS health journal at https://chucklinggoat.co.uk/gss/gss-health-journal.pdf

## Get in touch with me

Walking forward hand in hand, and sharing the information about natural healing that we discover as we go along – this is what it's all about, to me. I want to hear from you!

- To find inspiration: you can read more success stories from people who have already walked the GSS path here: https://chucklinggoat.co.uk/success-stories/

- To chat, share your own experience, opinions and thoughts, ask questions, and read our constantly updated stream of natural healing research and stories of life on the farm, you can find us here:

  **f**  **chucklinggoat**

  **𝕏**  **chucklinggoat**

  **◉**  **chucklinggoat**

- My blog site, where you can find more GSS recipes, info, hints, and tips, is **thefarmerswife.wales**

- You can contact me there, or email me at **info@chucklinggoat.co.uk**

I hope to be able to offer you a cup of tea someday, at our farmhouse kitchen table in Wales. If you're ever in the neighborhood, come and meet the goats.

Wishing you peace and strength on your way!

Hugs from the barn,

Shann

# References

## Chapter : Discoveries

1. Simpson C.R., Newton J., Hippisley-Cox J., Sheikh A. 'Trends in the epidemiology and prescribing of medication for eczema in England.' *Journal of the Royal Society of Medicine*, 2009; 102: 108-117

2. NHS Choices. 'Atopic Eczema.' Nov 11, 2014. www.nhs.uk/conditions/Eczema-(atopic)/Pages/Introduction.aspx

## Chapter 3: Heal the Gut, to Heal the Skin

1. University Of Dundee. 'New Findings Back Eczema Gene Link.' ScienceDaily. *ScienceDaily*, 26 September 2006. www.sciencedaily.com/releases/2006/09/060925080323.htm

2. https://nationaleczema.org/research/eczema-prevalence/

3. RIKEN. 'Genome-wide study identifies eight new susceptibility loci for atopic dermatitis.' ScienceDaily. *ScienceDaily*, 7 October 2012. www.sciencedaily.com/releases/2012/10/121007134829.htm

4. Schmitt J., Apfelbacher C.J., Flohr C. Eczema. *BMJ Clinical Evidence*. 2011; 2011:1716. www.ncbi.nlm.nih.gov/pmc/articles/PMC3217753/

5. National Eczema Association. 'Eczema prevalence in the United States.' www.nationaleczema.org/research/eczema-prevalence/

6. Ibid.

7. Wiley. 'No benefit of evening primrose oil for treating eczema, review suggests.' ScienceDaily. *ScienceDaily*, 29 April 2013. www.sciencedaily.com/releases/2013/04/130429210913.htm

8. The JAMA Network Journals. 'Symptoms of childhood eczema often persist a lifetime.' ScienceDaily *ScienceDaily*, 2 April 2014. www.sciencedaily.com/releases/2014/04/140402162452.htm

9. RIKEN. 'Genome-wide study identifies eight new susceptibility loci for atopic dermatitis.' ScienceDaily. *ScienceDaily*, 7 October 2012. www.sciencedaily.com/releases/2012/10/121007134829. htm

10. The JAMA Network Journals. 'Study quantifies costs, utilization, access to care for patients with eczema.' ScienceDaily. *ScienceDaily* 4 March 2015. www.sciencedaily.com/ releases/2015/03/150304124126.htm

11. LoBuono, C. 'For the First Time, Study Proves Eczema is an Autoimmune Disease.' Healthline News, 5 January 2015. www.healthline.com/health-news/study-proves-eczema-is-an-autoimmune-disease-010515#1

12. Guthrie, C. 'Autoimmune disorders: When your body turns on you.' *Experience Life*, October, 2013. www.experiencelife.com/ article/autoimmune-disorders-when-your-body-turns-on-you

13. Dotinga, R. 'More evidence of rosacea, autoimmune link.' *Dermatology Times*. April 7, 2016. www.dermatologytimes. modernmedicine.com/dermatology-times/news/more-evidence-rosacea-autoimmune-link

14. Cole, Dr. W. '12 Common triggers of autoimmune disease.' Mind Body Green. January 19, 2015. www.mindbodygreen.com/0-17100/12-common-triggers-of-autoimmune-disease.html

15. Guthrie, C. 'Autoimmune Disorders: When Your Body Turns on You.' *Experience Life*, October 2013. www.experiencelife.com/ article/autoimmune-disorders-when-your-body-turns-on-you

16. Helmholtz Centre For Environmental Research – UFZ. 'GI tract bacteria may protect against autoimmune disease.' ScienceDaily. *ScienceDaily*, 17 January 2013. www.sciencedaily.com/ releases/2013/01/130117133003.htm

17. Glynn, Sarah. 'Eczema Linked to Gut Bacteria in Kids.' *Medical News Today*, Wednesday 23 January 2013. www.medicalnewstoday. com/articles/255235

## Chapter 4: You Are a Superorganism!

1. Arizona State University. 'Clues about autism may come from the gut.' ScienceDaily. *ScienceDaily*, 4 July 2013. www.sciencedaily.com/releases/2013/07/130704095121.htm

2. University of Oxford. 'Competition between "good bacteria" important for healthy gut.' ScienceDaily. *ScienceDaily*, 5 November 2015. www.sciencedaily.com/releases/2015/11/151105152105.htm

3. University of Washington. 'Battle of the microbes: Pseudomonas breaches cell walls of rival bacteria without hurting itself.' ScienceDaily. *ScienceDaily*, 24 July 2011. www.sciencedaily.com/releases/2011/07/110720142129.htm

4. American Society for Microbiology. 'Humans Have Ten Times More Bacteria Than Human Cells: How Do Microbial Communities Affect Human Health?' ScienceDaily. *ScienceDaily*, 5 June 2008. www.sciencedaily.com/releases/2008/06/080603085914.htm

5. Vanderbilt University. 'Will the pronoun I become obsolete? A biological perspective.' ScienceDaily. *ScienceDaily*, 19 August 2015. www.sciencedaily.com/releases/2015/08/150819120658.htm

6. Oregon State University. 'Gut microbes closely linked to proper immune function, other health issues.' ScienceDaily. *ScienceDaily*, 16 September 2013. www.sciencedaily.com/releases/2013/09/130916122214.htm

## Chapter 5: Getting to Know Your Good Bugs

1. University of California, San Francisco (UCSF). 'Do gut bacteria rule our minds? In an ecosystem within us, microbes evolved to sway food choices.' ScienceDaily. *Science Daily*, 15 August 2014. www.sciencedaily.com/releases/2014/08/140815192240.htm

2. Cell Press. 'Gut microbes signal to the brain when they're full.' ScienceDaily. *ScienceDaily*, 24 November 2015. www.sciencedaily.com/releases/2015/11/151124143330.htm

3. University of California, San Francisco (UCSF). 'Do gut bacteria rule our minds? In an ecosystem within us, microbes evolved to sway food choices.' ScienceDaily. *ScienceDaily*, 15 August 2014. www.sciencedaily.com/releases/2014/08/140815192240.htm

4. California Institute of Technology. 'Learning to tolerate our microbial self: Bacteria co-opt human immune cells for mutual benefit.' ScienceDaily. *ScienceDaily*, 22 April 2011. www.sciencedaily.com/releases/2011/04/110421141632.htm

5. Ibid.

6. Ibid.

7. Ibid.

8. University of Michigan Health System. 'The Hygiene Hypothesis: Are Cleanlier Lifestyles Causing More Allergies For Kids?.' ScienceDaily. *ScienceDaily*, 9 September 2007. www.sciencedaily.com/releases/2007/09/070905174501.htm

9. London School of Hygiene & Tropical Medicine (LSHTM). 'Increase in allergies is not from being too clean, just losing touch with 'old friends'.' ScienceDaily. *ScienceDaily*, 3 October 2012. www.sciencedaily.com/releases/2012/10/121003082734.htm

10. Ibid.

11. Ibid.

## Chapter 6: Antibiotics and the Microbiome

1. Elsevier. 'Social media proves effective as a tool for antimicrobial stewardship." ScienceDaily. *ScienceDaily*, 31 October 2016. www.sciencedaily.com/releases/2016/10/161031124907.htm

2. Society for General Microbiology. 'Antibiotics have long-term impacts on gut flora.' ScienceDaily. *ScienceDaily*, 1 November 2010. www.sciencedaily.com/releases/2010/11/101101083144.htm

3. European Lung Foundation. 'Early life exposure to antibiotics is related to increased risk of allergies later in life.' ScienceDaily. *ScienceDaily*, 6 September 2016. www.sciencedaily.com/releases/2016/09/160906085003.htm

4. British Medical Journal (BMA). 'Harmful use of topical steroids in India is out of control, says expert.' ScienceDaily. *ScienceDaily*, 25 November 2015. www.sciencedaily.com/releases/2015/11/151125233022.htm

5. American Society for Microbiology. 'Antibiotics disrupt gut ecology, metabolism.' ScienceDaily. *ScienceDaily*, 20 April 2011. www.sciencedaily.com/releases/2011/04/110419214734.htm

6. Buhner, Stephen Harrod. *Herbal Antivirals: Natural Remedies for Emerging and Resistant Viral Infections.* North Adams: McNaughton and Gunn, Inc. 2013. p.11

7. UK government press release: 'Prime Minister warns of global threat of antibiotic resistance'. https://gov.uk/government/news/prime-minister-warns-of-global-threat-of-antibiotic-resistance

8. 'Antibiotic-resistant superbugs "will kill more than cancer" by 2050,' *The Week*, 11 December 2014, www.theweek.co.uk/51908/post-antibiotic-era-warning-after-gene-mutation-detected

9. Oregon State University. 'Unwanted impact of antibiotics broader, more complex than previously known.' ScienceDaily. *ScienceDaily*, 10 February 2015. www.sciencedaily.com/releases/2015/02/150210212634.htm

10. BioMed Central. 'Antibiotics Overprescribed By Doctors, Study Suggests.' ScienceDaily. *ScienceDaily*, 24 September 2007. www.sciencedaily.com/releases/2007/09/070920072119.htm

11. Infectious Diseases Society of America. 'Adverse Reactions To Antibiotics Send Thousands of Patients to the ER.' ScienceDaily. *ScienceDaily*, 13 August 2008. www.sciencedaily.com/releases/2008/08/080812135515.htm

12. Infectious Diseases Society of America. 'Antibiotics drastically overprescribed for sore throats, bronchitis.' ScienceDaily. *ScienceDaily*, 4 October 2013. www.sciencedaily.com/releases/2013/10/131004105256.htm

13. Oregon State University. 'Unwanted impact of antibiotics broader, more complex than previously known.' ScienceDaily. *ScienceDaily*, 10 February 2015. www.sciencedaily.com/releases/2015/02/150210212634.htm

14. Wyss Institute for Biologically Inspired Engineering at Harvard. 'New insights into how antibiotics damage human cells suggest novel strategies for making long-term antibiotic use safer.' ScienceDaily. *ScienceDaily*, 3 July 2013. www.sciencedaily.com/releases/2013/07/130703160623.htm

15. Oregon State University. 'Unwanted impact of antibiotics broader, more complex than previously known.' ScienceDaily. *ScienceDaily*, 10 February 2015. www.sciencedaily.com/releases/2015/02/150210212634.htm

16. University of Pennsylvania School of Medicine. 'Good' bacteria keep immune system primed to fight future infections.' ScienceDaily. *ScienceDaily*, 3 February 2010. www.sciencedaily. com/releases/2010/01/100127095945.htm

17. Ibid.

18. George Washington University. 'Patients don't understand risks of unnecessary antibiotics, study shows.' ScienceDaily. *ScienceDaily*, 15 December 2014. www.sciencedaily.com/ releases/2014/12/141215140857.htm

## Chapter 7: The Gut–Skin Connection

1. Perelman School of Medicine at the University of Pennsylvania. 'Immune system, skin microbiome "complement" one another.' ScienceDaily. *ScienceDaily*, 26 August 2013. www.sciencedaily. com/releases/2013/08/130826180513.htm

2. Johns Hopkins Medicine. 'Antibacterials in personal-care products linked to allergy risk in children.' ScienceDaily. *ScienceDaily*, 19 June 2012. www.sciencedaily.com/ releases/2012/06/120619092933.htm

3. Perelman School of Medicine at the University of Pennsylvania. 'Immune system, skin microbiome "complement" one another.' ScienceDaily. *ScienceDaily*, 26 August 2013. www.sciencedaily. com/releases/2013/08/130826180513.htm

4. NIH/National Institute of Allergy and Infectious Diseases. 'Protective role of skin microbiota described.' ScienceDaily. *ScienceDaily*, 26 July 2012. www.sciencedaily.com/ releases/2012/07/120726153947.htm

5. Perelman School of Medicine at the University of Pennsylvania. 'Immune system, skin microbiome "complement" one another.' ScienceDaily. *ScienceDaily*, 26 August 2013. www.sciencedaily. com/releases/2013/08/130826180513.htm

6. Arizona State University. 'War and peace in the human gut: Probing the microbiome.' ScienceDaily. *ScienceDaily*, 6 June 2016. www.sciencedaily.com/releases/2016/06/160606200431.htm

7. University of Guelph. 'Link between stress, unhealthy microbiomes discovered.' ScienceDaily. *ScienceDaily*, 6 January 2016. www.sciencedaily.com/releases/2016/01/ 160106091735.htm

8.  Oregon State University. 'Common antimicrobial agent rapidly disrupts gut bacteria.' ScienceDaily. *ScienceDaily*, 18 May 2016. www.sciencedaily.com/releases/2016/05/160518152805.htm

9.  University of Michigan. 'Antibacterial soaps: Being too clean can make people sick, study suggests.' ScienceDaily. *ScienceDaily*, 30 November 2010. www.sciencedaily.com/releases/2010/11/101129101920.htm

10. 'Superbug Threat is Ticking Time Bomb.' NHS Choices. 11 March 2013. www.nhs.uk/news/2013/03March/Pages/Superbug-threat-is-ticking-time-bomb.aspx

11. University College London. 'Could Plain Soap And Probiotics Beat Hospital Bugs?' ScienceDaily. *ScienceDaily*, 31 October 2005. www.sciencedaily.com/releases/2005/10/051031132130.htm

12. BioMed Central Limited. 'Eczema in infants linked to gut bacteria.' ScienceDaily. *ScienceDaily*, 23 January 2013. www.sciencedaily.com/releases/2013/01/130122231351.htm

13. NYU Langone Medical Center / New York University School of Medicine. 'Intestinal bacteria linked to rheumatoid arthritis.' ScienceDaily. *ScienceDaily*, 5 November 2013. www.sciencedaily.com/releases/2013/11/131105132031.htm

14. Technical University of Munich (TUM). 'Intestinal bacteria influence food allergies: Composition of gut microbiota and immune system are closely interwoven.' ScienceDaily. *ScienceDaily*, 7 September 2016. www.sciencedaily.com/releases/2016/09/160907125125.htm

15. Cedars-Sinai Medical Center. 'Irritable bowel syndrome clearly linked to gut bacteria.' ScienceDaily. *ScienceDaily*, 25 May 2012. www.sciencedaily.com/releases/2012/05/120525103354.htm

16. Columbia University's Mailman School of Public Health. 'Robust evidence that chronic fatigue syndrome is a biological illness.' ScienceDaily. *ScienceDaily*, 27 February 2015. www.sciencedaily.com/releases/2015/02/150227144903.htm

17. California Institute of Technology. 'Of bugs and brains: Gut bacteria affect multiple sclerosis.' ScienceDaily. *ScienceDaily*, 20 July 2010. www.sciencedaily.com/releases/2010/07/100719162643.htm

18. Institut Pasteur. 'Role of microbiota in preventing allergies.' ScienceDaily. *ScienceDaily*, 10 July 2015. www.sciencedaily.com/releases/2015/07/150710095244.htm

19. University of Helsinki. 'Biodiversity loss may cause increase in allergies and asthma.' ScienceDaily. *ScienceDaily*, 7 May 2012. www.sciencedaily.com/releases/2012/05/120507154114.htm

20. McMaster University. 'Link between intestinal bacteria, depression found.' ScienceDaily. *ScienceDaily*, 28 July 2015. www.sciencedaily.com/releases/2015/07/150728110734.htm

21. University of Michigan. 'Antibacterial soaps: Being too clean can make people sick, study suggests.' ScienceDaily. *ScienceDaily*, 30 November 2010. www.sciencedaily.com/releases/2010/11/101129101920.htm

22. University College London. 'Could Plain Soap And Probiotics Beat Hospital Bugs?' ScienceDaily. *ScienceDaily*, 31 October 2005. www.sciencedaily.com/releases/2005/10/051031132130.htm

23. Oregon State University. 'Unwanted impact of antibiotics broader, more complex than previously known.' ScienceDaily. *ScienceDaily*, 10 February 2015. www.sciencedaily.com/releases/2015/02/150210212634.htm

## Chapter 8: Eczema and Allergic Disease

1. University of Melbourne. 'Childhood eczema and hay fever leads to adult allergic asthma, study finds.' ScienceDaily. *ScienceDaily*, 15 April 2011. www.sciencedaily.com/releases/2011/04/110415104534.htm

2. Rush University Medical Center. 'Allergic Disease Linked To Irritable Bowel Syndrome.' ScienceDaily. *ScienceDaily*, 31 January 2008. www.sciencedaily.com/releases/2008/01/080130170325.htm

3. European Academy of Allergology and Clinical Immunology (EAACI). 'Breastfeeding reduces the risk of allergies, study suggests.' ScienceDaily. *ScienceDaily*, 14 October 2011. www.sciencedaily.com/releases/2011/10/111014104404.htm

4. Deutsche Gesellschaft fuer Immunologie e.V./German Society for Immunology. 'Allergy: Solving The Mystery Of IgE.' ScienceDaily. *ScienceDaily*, 14 September 2009. www.sciencedaily.com/releases/2009/09/090914111537.htm

5. European Academy of Allergology and Clinical Immunology (EAACI). 'Breastfeeding reduces the risk of allergies, study suggests.' ScienceDaily. *ScienceDaily*, 14 October 2011. www.sciencedaily.com/releases/2011/10/111014104404.htm

6.  Ohio State University. 'Hay Fever Can Send Work Productivity Down The Drain.' ScienceDaily. *ScienceDaily*, 26 April 2007. www.sciencedaily.com/releases/2007/04/070426093436.htm

7.  Virginia Commonwealth University. 'Key Molecular Signaling Switch Involved In Allergic Disease Identified.' ScienceDaily. *ScienceDaily*, 30 October 2006. www.sciencedaily.com/releases/2006/10/061029174930.htm

8.  American Academy of Dermatology (AAD). 'Dermatologists caution that atopic dermatitis is a strong precursor to food allergies.' ScienceDaily. *ScienceDaily*, 7 February 2011. www.sciencedaily.com/releases/2011/02/110205140828.htm

9.  University of Melbourne. 'Childhood eczema and hay fever leads to adult allergic asthma, study finds.' ScienceDaily. *ScienceDaily*, 15 April 2011. www.sciencedaily.com/releases/2011/04/110415104534.htm

10. Washington University School of Medicine. 'Why Eczema Often Leads to Asthma.' ScienceDaily. *ScienceDaily*, 20 May 2009. www.sciencedaily.com/releases/2009/05/090518213939.htm

11. University of Melbourne. 'Childhood eczema and hay fever leads to adult allergic asthma, study finds.' ScienceDaily. *ScienceDaily*, 15 April 2011. www.sciencedaily.com/releases/2011/04/110415104534.htm

12. University of Pennsylvania School of Medicine. 'Border patrol: Immune cells protect body from invaders.' ScienceDaily. *ScienceDaily*, 9 February 2011. www.sciencedaily.com/releases/2011/02/110207142621.htm

13. University of Rochester Medical Center. 'Major shift in understanding how eczema develops.' ScienceDaily. *ScienceDaily*, 18 December 2010. www.sciencedaily.com/releases/2010/12/101217145920.htm

14. Ibid.

15. Ibid.

## Chapter 9: Adventures Inside Your Immune System

1.  Washington University School of Medicine. 'Why Eczema Often Leads to Asthma.' ScienceDaily. *ScienceDaily*, 20 May 2009. www.sciencedaily.com/releases/2009/05/090518213939.htm

2. Oregon State University. 'Researchers discover genetic basis for eczema, new avenue to therapies.' ScienceDaily. *ScienceDaily*, 21 December 2012. www.sciencedaily.com/releases/2012/12/121221131259.htm

3. Washington University School of Medicine. 'Why Eczema Often Leads To Asthma.' ScienceDaily. *ScienceDaily*, 20 May 2009. www.sciencedaily.com/releases/2009/05/090518213939.htm

4. Ibid.

5. University of California – Berkeley. 'Blocking nerve cells could prevent symptoms of eczema.' ScienceDaily. *ScienceDaily*, 3 October 2013. www.sciencedaily.com/releases/2013/10/131003121300.htm

6. Washington University School of Medicine. 'Why Eczema Often Leads to Asthma.' ScienceDaily. *ScienceDaily*, 20 May 2009. www.sciencedaily.com/releases/2009/05/090518213939.htm

7. University of Pennsylvania School of Medicine. 'Slowing the allergic march.' ScienceDaily. *ScienceDaily*, 16 August 2011. www.sciencedaily.com/releases/2011/08/110814141508.htm

8. NIH/National Institute of Allergy and Infectious Diseases. 'Switch turns on allergic disease in people.' ScienceDaily. *ScienceDaily*, 22 January 2010. www.sciencedaily.com/releases/2010/01/100120144003.htm

9. Washington University in St. Louis. 'Skin Defects Set Off Alarm With Widespread and Potentially Harmful Effects.' ScienceDaily. *ScienceDaily*, 1 June 2008. www.sciencedaily.com/releases/2008/05/080527201755.htm

10. McMaster University. 'New potential antibody treatment for asthma discovered.' ScienceDaily. *ScienceDaily*, 20 May 2014. www.sciencedaily.com/releases/2014/05/140520122957.htm

11. Helmholtz Zentrum Muenchen – German Research Centre for Environmental Health. 'Key Allergy Gene Discovered.' ScienceDaily. *ScienceDaily*, 25 August 2008. www.sciencedaily.com/releases/2008/08/080822085111.htm

12. Austrian Science Fund. 'High Levels Of Antibodies, Low Levels Of Cancer?' ScienceDaily. *ScienceDaily*, 17 April 2007. www.sciencedaily.com/releases/2007/04/070416170327.htm

## Chapter 10: Psoriasis, Rosacea, and Acne

1. Health Union. 'Plaque psoriasis patients find many treatments, but few satisfied with their current plan: National survey finds many wish they would have known impact psoriasis would have on their mental and physical health.' ScienceDaily. *ScienceDaily*, 16 August 2016. www.sciencedaily.com/releases/2016/08/160816092213.htm

2. American Academy of Dermatology. 'Psoriasis is more than skin deep.' ScienceDaily. *ScienceDaily*, 6 March 2010. www.sciencedaily.com/releases/2010/03/100306104436.htm

3. Hokkaido University. 'Understanding the underlying mechanisms that lead to psoriasis.' ScienceDaily. ScienceDaily, 25 May 2016. www.sciencedaily.com/releases/2016/05/160525084539.htm

4. Adiloglu, A.K. 'The effect of kefir on human immune system: a cytokine study.' United National Library of Medicine. National Institutes of Health. April 2013. www.ncbi.nlm.nih.gov/pubmed/23621727.

5. Society for Neuroscience. 'How Inflammatory Disease Causes Fatigue.' ScienceDaily. *ScienceDaily*, 28 February 2009. www.sciencedaily.com/releases/2009/02/090217173034.htm

6. Dotinga, R. 'More evidence of rosacea, autoimmune link.' Dermatology Times. April 7, 2016. www.dermatologytimes.modernmedicine.com/dermatology-times/news/more-evidence-rosacea-autoimmune-link.

7. Society for General Microbiology. 'Bacterial cause found for skin condition rosacea.' ScienceDaily. *ScienceDaily*, 29 August 2012. www.sciencedaily.com/releases/2012/08/120829195121.htm

8. University of California, San Diego. 'Cause of Skin Condition Rosacea Discovered.' ScienceDaily. *ScienceDaily*, 7 August 2007. www.sciencedaily.com/releases/2007/08/070805161110.htm

9. Sturgis, I. 'The rise of adult acne is like an epidemic.' *The Telegraph*: Lifestyle: Wellbeing. January 18, 2016. www.telegraph.co.uk/wellbeing/health-advice/the-rise-of-adult-acne-is-like-an-epidemic/

10. Muszer, M., et al. 'Human Microbiome: When a Friend Becomes an Enemy.' Archivum Immunologiae et Therapiae Experimentalis 63.4 (2015): 287–298. PMC. Web. 12 Nov 2016. www.ncbi.nlm.nih.gov/pubmed/25682593.

11. Sturgis, 'I. The rise of adult acne is like an epidemic.' *The Telegraph*: Lifestyle: Wellbeing. January 18, 2016. www.telegraph.co.uk/wellbeing/health-advice/the-rise-of-adult-acne-is-like-an-epidemic

12. Ibid.

13. Ibid.

14. American Academy of Dermatology. 'Feeling Stressed? How Your Skin, Hair and Nails Can Show It.' ScienceDaily. *ScienceDaily*, 12 November 2007. www.sciencedaily.com/releases/2007/11/071109194053.htm

15. University of California, Los Angeles (UCLA), Health Sciences. 'Why some people get zits and others don't.' ScienceDaily. *ScienceDaily*, 28 February 2013. www.sciencedaily.com/releases/2013/02/130228080135.htm

16. Canadian Medical Association Journal. 'Birth defects, pregnancy terminations, miscarriages in users of acne drug.' ScienceDaily. *ScienceDaily*, 25 April 2016. www.sciencedaily.com/releases/2016/04/160425141528.htm

17. Journal of Investigative Dermatology. 'Propionibacterium acnes Strain Populations in the Human Skin Microbiome Associated with Acne.' September 2013. Volume 133, Issue 9, pages 2152–2160

18. Thyme may be better for acne than prescription creams. www.microbiologysociety.org/news/press-releases.cfm/thyme-may-be-better-for-acne-than-prescription-creams

19. University College Cork. 'Mind-altering microbes: Probiotic bacteria may lessen anxiety and depression.' ScienceDaily. *ScienceDaily*, 30 August 2011. www.sciencedaily.com/releases/2011/08/110829164601.htm

20. American Academy of Dermatology. 'What to Eat for Glowing Healthy Skin.' ScienceDaily. *ScienceDaily*, 15 November 2007. www.sciencedaily.com/releases/2007/11/071109201438.htm

## Chapter 11: Kefir: A Probiotic Powerhouse

1. Society of Chemical Industry. 'Friendly Bacteria in Alcoholic Milkshake Could Fight Food Allergies.' ScienceDaily. *ScienceDaily*, 16 October 2006. www.sciencedaily.com/releases/2006/10/061015213714.htm

2. Ibid.

3. Hong, Wei-Sheng. 'The Antiallergic Effect of Kefir Lactobacilli.' Health Nutrition and Food. Journal of Food Science, Volume 75, Issue 8, October 2010.

4. American Society for Microbiology. 'Dairy products boost effectiveness of probiotics.' ScienceDaily. *ScienceDaily*, 17 July 2015. www.sciencedaily.com/releases/2015/07/150717142439.htm

5. University of Granada. 'Goats' Milk Is More Beneficial to Health Than Cows' Milk, Study Suggests.' ScienceDaily. *ScienceDaily*, 31 July 2007. www.sciencedaily.com/releases/2007/07/070730100229.htm

6. Albert Einstein College of Medicine. 'Probiotics May Help People Taking Antibiotics.' ScienceDaily. *ScienceDaily*, 24 December 2008. www.sciencedaily.com/releases/2008/12/081217190443.htm

## Chapter 14: GSS Habit #1: Drink Goat's Milk Kefir

1. University of Bristol. 'Lactate and brain function: How the body regulates fundamental neuro-hormone.' ScienceDaily. *ScienceDaily*, 11 February 2014. www.sciencedaily.com/releases/2014/02/140211084053.htm

2. Kalia, S. 'Why You Should Drink Kefir Even if You're Lactose-Intolerant.' FitLife.tv. Feb 26, 2015. www.fitlife.tv/why-you-should-drink-kefir-even-if-youre-lactose-intolerant_original/

3. Marco, Mariángeles Briggiler. Bacteriophages and dairy fermentations. Journal List. US National Library of Medicine. National Institutes of Health. June 2012. www.ncbi.nlm.nih.gov/pmc/articles/PMC3530524/

4. Norwegian School of Veterinary Science. 'Viruses Can Turn Harmless E. Coli Dangerous.' ScienceDaily. *ScienceDaily*, 22 April 2009. www.sciencedaily.com/releases/2009/04/090417195827.htm

## Chapter 15: GSS Habit #2: Use Goat's Milk Kefir Skincare

1. Rice, M. 'Revealed... the 515 chemicals women put on their bodies every day.' *Daily Mail.* Beauty. Nov 21, 2009. www. dailymail.co.uk/femail/beauty/article–1229275/Revealed–-515-chemicals-women-bodies-day.html

2. Guthrie, C. 'Autoimmune Disorders: When Your Body Turns on You.' *Experience Life.* Oct 2013. www.experiencelife.com/article/autoimmune-disorders-when-your-body-turns-on-you

3. National Eczema Organization, UK. www.nationaleczema.org/ education-announcement-topical-corticosteroids-eczema/

4. Lucia, F. 'B.C. Woman Whose Skin Fell Off Warns About Steroid Addiction.' Huffington Post B.C. May 15, 2015. www.huffingtonpost.ca/2015/05/15/steroid-cream-addiction_n_7236986.html

5. American Academy of Dermatology. 'Could probiotics be the next big thing in acne and rosacea treatments?' Jan 30, 2014. www.aad.org/media/news-releases/could-probiotics-be-the-next-big-thing-in-acne-and-rosacea-treatments

## Chapter 17: GSS Habit #4: Replace Sugar with Stevia

1. Verburgh, Dr. K. *The Food Hourglass,* London: Harper Collins, 2014, page 50

2. Goyal, S.K. 'Stevia (Stevia rebaudiana) a bio-sweetener: a review.' www.ncbi.nlm.nih.gov/pubmed/19961353, Feb 2010

3. Jockers, D. 'Stevia is a natural anti-inflammatory and anti-cancer agent.' Natural News, www.naturalnews.com/048909_stevia_ natural_anti-inflammatory_anti-cancer.html, March 8, 2015

4. Goyal, S.K. 'Stevia (Stevia rebaudiana) a bio-sweetener: a review.' www.ncbi.nlm.nih.gov/pubmed/19961353, Feb 2010

5. NHS Choices. 'Can Honey Fight Superbugs like MRSA?' www. nhs.uk/news/2011/04April/Pages/manuka-honey-mrsa-superbug-bacteria.aspx, Apr 13, 2011

6. Morgan, M. 'Is your superfood honey FAKE? Experts reveal that three times more jars of healing manuka are sold around the

world than being produced in New Zealand,' Daily Mail, www.dailymail.co.uk/femail/article-3066381/Is-superfood-honey-FAKE-jars-manuka-sold-world-produced-New-Zealand.html, May 3, 2015

7. 'Scottish honey 'is as good at healing as manuka': Heather variety could offer cheaper alternative,' Daily Mail, www.dailymail.co.uk/health/article-2440926/Scottish-honey-good-healing-manuka-Heather-variety-offer-cheaper-alternative.html#ixzz4AiVVJXiU, Oct 2, 2013

## Chapter 18: GSS Habit #5: Eat Goat Dairy

1. University of Granada. 'Goat milk can be considered as functional food, Spanish researchers find.' ScienceDaily. *ScienceDaily*, 19 May 2011. www.sciencedaily.com/releases/2011/05/110518092146.htm

2. Olivier, C.E. et al. 'Is It Just Lactose Intolerance?,' Allergy Asthma Proc. Sept–Oct 2012. /www.ncbi.nlm.nih.gov/pubmed/23026186.

3. University of Granada. 'Goat milk can be considered as functional food, Spanish researchers find.' ScienceDaily. *ScienceDaily*, 19 May 2011. www.sciencedaily.com/releases/2011/05/110518092146.htm

4. University of Granada. 'Goats' milk is more beneficial to health than cows' milk, study suggests.' ScienceDaily. *ScienceDaily*, 31 July 2007. www.sciencedaily.com/releases/2007/07/070730100229.htm

5. University of Granada. 'Goat milk can be considered as functional food, Spanish researchers find.' ScienceDaily. *ScienceDaily*, 19 May 2011. www.sciencedaily.com/releases/2011/05/110518092146.htm

6. Ibid.

7. Ibid

8. Ibid.

9. Ibid

## Chapter 19: GSS Habit #6: Choose Slow-Burning Foods

1.  Fred Hutchinson Cancer Research Center. 'Diet rich in slowly digested carbs reduces markers of inflammation in overweight and obese adults.' ScienceDaily. *ScienceDaily*, 12 January 2012. www.sciencedaily.com/releases/2012/01/120111154043.htm

## Chapter 20: GSS Habit #7: Go for Good Fats

1.  McMaster University. 'Trans fats, but not saturated fats like butter, linked to greater risk of early death and heart disease.' ScienceDaily. *ScienceDaily*, 11 August 2015. www.sciencedaily.com/releases/2015/08/150811215545.htm

2.  'Butter leads to lower blood fats than olive oil, study finds.' ScienceDaily. *ScienceDaily*, 10 February 2010. www.sciencedaily.com/releases/2010/02/100209124352.htm

3.  American Chemical Society. 'New piece in the 'French paradox' diet and health puzzle: Cheese metabolism.' ScienceDaily. *ScienceDaily*, 8 April 2015. www.sciencedaily.com/releases/2015/04/150408124618.htm

4.  University of Alberta. 'Eggs' antioxidant properties may help prevent heart disease and cancer, study suggests.' ScienceDaily. *ScienceDaily*, 6 July 2011. www.sciencedaily.com/releases/2011/07/110706093900.htm

5.  Axe, Dr. J. 'Budwig Diet Protocol for Cancer.' www.draxe.com/budwig-diet-protocol-cancer/.

6.  Canadian Science Publishing (NRC Research Press). 'Beating high blood pressure with a combination of coconut oil and physical exercise: Animal study.' ScienceDaily. *ScienceDaily*, 9 February 2015. www.sciencedaily.com/releases/2015/02/150209171317.htm

7.  Tufts University, Health Sciences Campus. 'Coconut oil can control overgrowth of a fungal pathogen in GI tract, study in mice suggests.' ScienceDaily. *ScienceDaily*, 18 November 2015. www.sciencedaily.com/releases/2015/11/151118125325.htm

8.  University of California, San Diego. 'Treat acne with coconut oil and nano-bombs.' ScienceDaily. *ScienceDaily*, 15 April 2010. www.sciencedaily.com/releases/2010/04/100414184224.htm

9.  Agero, A.L. 'A randomized double-blind controlled trial comparing extra virgin coconut oil with mineral oil as a moisturizer for mild

to moderate xerosis.' *Dermatitis*. September 15, 2004. www.ncbi. nlm.nih.gov/pubmed/15724344.

10. Society for General Microbiology. 'Coconut oil could combat tooth decay.' ScienceDaily. *ScienceDaily*, 2 September 2012. www. sciencedaily.com/releases/2012/09/120902222459.htm

11. 'The Top 4 Avocado Skin Benefits,' Healthiest Foods. www. healthiestfoods.co.uk/avocado-skin-benefits.

12. Penn State. 'Walnuts, walnut oil, improve reaction to stress.' ScienceDaily. *ScienceDaily*, 4 October 2010. www.sciencedaily. com/releases/2010/10/101004101141.htm

## Conclusion: Three Essential Lessons

1. Loyola University Health System. 'Boost your immune system, shake off stress by walking in the woods.' ScienceDaily. *ScienceDaily*, 3 October 2013. www.sciencedaily.com/releases/ 2013/10/131003132112.htm

2. Ibid.

3. Ibid.

4. University of Eastern Finland. "Early childhood exposure to farm animals, pets modifies immunological responses." ScienceDaily. *ScienceDaily*, 14 December 2015. www.sciencedaily.com/ releases/2015/12/151214085004.htm

5. Aarhus University. 'The immune system benefits from life in the countryside.' ScienceDaily. ScienceDaily, 30 September 2013. www.sciencedaily.com/releases/2013/09/130930101841.htm

6. Ibid.

7. Ibid.

8. Massachusetts General Hospital. 'Vitamin D significantly improves symptoms of winter-related atopic dermatitis in children.' ScienceDaily. *ScienceDaily*, 3 October 2014. www. sciencedaily.com/releases/2014/10/141003135423.htm

# Suggested Reading

Here are just a few of the favorite books I keep close at hand on my shelf:

*The Allergy Solution: Unlock the Surprising, Hidden Truth about Why You Are Sick and How to Get Well*, Dr. Leo Galland and Jonathan Galland (Hay House, 2016)

*The Art of Fermentation: An In-depth Exploration of Essential Concepts and Processes from Around the World*, Sandor Ellix Katz (Chelsea Green Publishing, 2012)

*The Bone Broth Secret: A Culinary Adventure in Health, Beauty, and Longevity*, Louise Hay and Heather Dane (Hay House, 2016)

*Brain Maker: The Power of Gut Microbes to Heal and Protect Your Brain – for Life*, David Perlmutter (Little, Brown Book Group, 2015)

*The Complete Farmhouse Cookbook.* Mary Norwak and Baby Honey (Michael Russell Publishing, 1973)

*The Food Hourglass: Stay Younger for Longer and Lose Weight*, Kris Verburgh (Harper Collins, 2014)

*Gut and Psychology Syndrome: Natural Treatment for Autism, Dyspraxia, A.D.D., Dyslexia, A.D.H.D., Depression, Schizophrenia*, Dr. Natasha Campbell-McBride (Medinform Publishing, 2004)

*Look Great Naturally... Without Ditching the Lipstick*, Janey Lee Grace (Hay House, 2013)

*Nourishing Traditions: The Cookbook that Challenges Politically Correct Nutrition and Diet Dictocrats*, Sally Fallon (New Trends Publishing; 2nd revised edition, 2001)

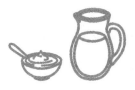

# Resources

## Goat's milk kefir

Chuckling's Goat's drinking kefir is made with goat's milk and real kefir grains, and left pure and unflavored for maximum potency. Our kefir is made by hand in small batches, and demand is high, so there may be a queue.

It can be shipped to your door anywhere inside the UK. Unfortunately we are unable to ship our kefir abroad, because of the restrictions on shipping liquids. Our kefir grains are proprietary and registered to the farm, and are not for sale.

## Goat's milk kefir skincare

Chucking Goat's kefir skincare begins with a base of our own kefir and goat's milk, produced here on the farm. The goat's milk is anti-inflammatory and penetrates the barrier of the human skin, carrying its load of vitamins and minerals, while the probiotic kefir re-populates the good bacteria in the skin biome.

To this base, we then add a variety of essential oils, each of which produces a different effect (two ranges contain no oils).

We've created five skincare ranges to meet our clients' needs. Each has a cleansing bar, a lotion, and a bath melt.

- **Break-Out** – with thyme and tea tree essential oils

- **Soothing** – with rosemary essential oil

- **Calm-Down** – with lavender essential oil

- **Sensitive** – without essential oil

- **Baby** – without essential oil; suitable for infants from one month

Our skincare is suitable for all skin conditions, including eczema, psoriasis, rosacea, and acne. The main variance in the ranges is the difference in strength.

Break-Out is our most powerful and quickest-acting formulation, followed by Soothing, Calm-Down, Sensitive and then Baby – our gentlest formulation designed specifically for delicate, baby skin.

### Eczema, psoriasis, rosacea, and acne

We always recommend our Break-Out range to help combat these skin issues. This is our strongest formulation, and as long as the client doesn't have an allergy to thyme or tea tree essential oils, and/or doesn't have particularly sensitive skin, it's the perfect skincare for them.

The essential oils may sting broken skin, so I advise avoiding those areas. Or opt for the next range down. If you'd like to use one skincare product alone, I always strongly recommend the lotion above all others, as we've had the best results with this particular product. You can apply the lotion as often as you like – there's nothing in there that will harm the skin. Bath melts are handy for skin issues that occur over the entire body.

Break-Out is age tested 12+, as thyme and tea tree are strong essential oils. It can be used on children under the age of 12 at parents' discretion. We suggest that you perform a small patch test on the inside of the wrist; if there's no redness or stinging within 10 minutes, the lotion and cleanser is safe to use.

## Hives, rashes, and inflamed skin

For inflammation or red/hot skin issues, we tend to suggest the Soothing range. The rosemary essential oil it contains has natural anti-inflammatory properties that reduce redness and alleviate irritation. Soothing bath melts and Soothing lotion are highly recommended for all-over skin issues.

## Sensitive skin/children under the age of 12

The Sensitive range is suitable for those with super-sensitive skin, and for children under the age of 12 (it is age tested 3+).

This range contains no essential oils, just oatmeal, honey, kefir, goat's milk and Finnish oat oil, so it's super soft and gentle. Some clients opt for the Calm-Down range, which is essentially the notch up from Sensitive. The cleansing bar can be used in the shower – which helps clients' avoid using shower gels that contain perfumes and chemicals.

## Dry skin

I usually advise the use of either the Calm-Down or Sensitive ranges in these instances. Calm-Down contains lavender essential oil, which has some antibacterial properties as well as being very gentle. As it's quite a mild essential oil, it doesn't dry out the skin and leaves it feeling super smooth.

## Infant skin conditions

For babies and toddlers we always suggest the use of our Baby range. This is our simplest, purest formulation and has no fragrance, perfumes, or essential oils. It's age tested from one month to 3 years, so is completely safe to use on little ones. Baby Bath Melts are perfect for babies as they're bathed often.

## Pregnancy

Our Sensitive range contains the most appropriate products for use during pregnancy, as pregnant women are recommended to avoid all essential oils.

# Giving Thanks

I have been so very fortunate in my life. I'm deeply grateful both for the crises that have taught me so much, and the good fortune that has carried me through them.

Most of all, I'm grateful for the people around me. My wholehearted thanks go out to:

**Louise Hay**, who created a publishing house that's one of the most amazing things I've ever encountered. Louise Hay and her team at Hay House really do walk their talk, in the mind-body-spirit world. They are real, genuine, inspired and inspiring, heart-motivated, and looking to push humanity forward. I am blessed to be included in the very happy family of Hay House authors!

**Reid Tracey**, who first saw the potential in my little diary and our tiny business. He published one, and invested in the other, allowing us to thrive and grow. Without Reid, none of this would have happened. Thank you for having faith in us when no one else did!

**Michelle Pilley**, whose wisdom, warmth, and lucid vision helped it all come together. To be the recipient of your guidance is a lovely thing.

**Julie Oughton**, who edits with a skill and generosity that make it a pleasure to be edited... who knew? Lucky me, to have your fine brain focused on my crazy heap of ideas and drag them into some sort of lucid structure.

**Debra Wolter**, whose incredibly detailed, patient and thorough line edit should really earn her a co-writing credit. Above and beyond the call of duty, Debra, thank you so much for all your hard work and patience!! The good bugs love you.

**Jo Burgess and Sian Orrell**, those queens of marketing who raise it to a fine art – and make it all fun, to boot. Great to have such savvy mixed with such authentic loveliness. All your help getting the message out is deeply appreciated.

**Diane Hill**, who expertly deals with sales and the mad American side of things, and never loses her sense of humor.

**Leanne Siu Anastasi**, who was incredibly patient with my ditherings, understood what I was on about, and nailed it in the end... twice! Thanks, Leanne.

**Tom Cole**, whose technical brilliance and social marketing expertise makes him an unending source of incredibly useful information. Tom, you make it look easy!

And all the rest of the cast and crew at Hay House. The goats love you guys!

**Janey Lee Grace**, who loved our products, mentored me, and convinced me that I really should write a book. Just look what you've started, Janey! Couldn't have done it without you – thank you for fanning the flames of our little endeavor.

Deepest gratitude also to:

**Bonnie Nadell**, the agent who has stuck with me for almost 30 years now, through all the ups and downs, of which – ahem – there have been many. Always brilliant, and professional to her fingertips. Thanks for your faith and loyalty, Bonnie – much appreciated!

And of course, my beloved family:

**My husband Rich**, who has saved me in every way that one person can save another. You took on a mad American and civilized her when no one thought it could be done. Love you forever.

**Our deeply cherished children:** Ceris, Elly, Joli, and Benj – partners George and Josh – and our grandson Macsen! All of you are always in my heart. Being surrounded by you makes me happy, and that means everything to me.

**To my mother Ann**, who has forgiven me for making so many mistakes in my life, and still loves me anyway! Thanks for sticking with me on the long and bumpy journey – and for chanting and drumming as I walk my road.

**To my father, Don**, who so generously supported us during our rocky time.

**And last but not least, my beloved goats.** Everything I really needed to know, they taught me, in the end.

# ABOUT THE AUTHOR

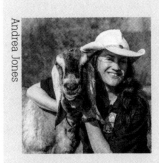

Andrea Jones

**Shann Nix Jones** was the ultimate American city girl until she fell in love with a Welsh farmer at the age of 41. Shann and her husband, Rich, realized that they could do something extraordinary when they started to work with goats' milk and used it to heal their son's eczema, and Rich's life-threatening superbug infection. They decided to quit their respective day jobs, and try to make a go of the goats'-milk business full time. They now have 70 goats who have become like members of the family.

In April 2011, the couple launched their online business, Chuckling Goat, selling health-enhancing soaps, creams and probiotic kefir drinks, which they make by hand on the farm. The launch was a huge success, and today their award-winning homemade products are available all over the United Kingdom.

**f** chucklinggoat

**🐦** chucklinggoat

**📷** chucklinggoat

**✉** info@chucklinggoat.co.uk

**www.chucklinggoat.co.uk**

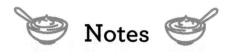

# Notes

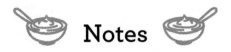 **Notes**

# HAY HOUSE
## *Look within*

Join the conversation about latest products,
events, exclusive offers and more.

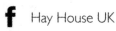 Hay House UK

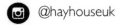 @HayHouseUK

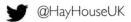 @hayhouseuk

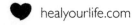 healyourlife.com

*We'd love to hear from you!*